HOUSE CALLS AROUND THE WORLD

A GLOBAL MEDICAL ADVENTURE

Charles B. Sherman, MD, MPH, DGM

House Calls Around the World: A Global Medical Adventure
Copyright © 2021 Charles B. Sherman, MD, MPH, DGM

Produced and printed by Stillwater River Publications.
All rights reserved. Written and produced in the United States of America. This book may not be reproduced or sold in any form without the expressed, written permission of the author(s) and publisher.

Visit our website at **www.StillwaterPress.com** for more information.

First Stillwater River Publications Edition

ISBN: 978-1-955123-52-5

Library of Congress Control Number: 2021919455

Photo of Tolyatti, Russia by Mstyslav Chernov, via Wikimedia Commons.
Photo of Basotho women by VirtualSteve, via Wikimedia Commons.
Photo of gelada baboon by Tambako The Jaguar on Flickr.
Photo of fresco at Abuna Yemata Guh uploaded to Flickr by Owen Barder.

2 3 4 5 6 7 8 9 10
Written by Charles B. Sherman, MD, MPH, DGM
Published by Stillwater River Publications, Pawtucket, RI, USA.

Publisher's Cataloging-In-Publication Data
(Prepared by The Donohue Group, Inc.)

Names: Sherman, Charles B., 1954- author.
Title: House calls around the world : a global medical adventure / Charles B. Sherman, MD, MPH, DGM.
Description: First Stillwater River Publications edition. | Pawtucket, RI, USA : Stillwater River Publications, [2021]
Identifiers: ISBN 9781955123525
Subjects: LCSH: Sherman, Charles B.--Travel. | Physicians--United States--Biography. | World health--20th century. | World health--21st century. | LCGFT: Autobiographies.
Classification: LCC R154.S456 A3 2021 | DDC 610.92--dc23

The views and opinions expressed in this book are solely those of the author(s) and do not necessarily reflect the views and opinions of the publisher.

*For those who matter most: Kathie and the Ducks
(Steve, Glenn, Rafi, Lev, Phoebe, Mya, Gianni, and Nico).*

November 10, 2024

"Travel is kinship to humanity."
—*Ibn Battuta, 14th century Moroccan explorer*

"It's not what one lived but how one remembers it."
—*Gabriel Garcia Marquez*

CONTENTS

Preface .... *ix*

1	Take Two Aspirin	1
2	Stay Right There	5
3	The World's Worst Hospital Orderly	14
4	I Can't See	19
5	Smile	26
6	It Was a Dark and Stormy Night	34
7	The CIA Plot	42
8	To Learn to Truly Fly	51
9	Director of Good Moments	55
10	The Flying Nun	62
11	Building the Runway	67
12	You Want Me to Do What?	73
13	Dirt Nap	81

Acknowledgements 86
About the Author 87

PREFACE

I wrote this collection of stories after I had finally retired from the clinical practice of medicine. Writing has always been the best way for me to explore my feelings. So, with more time on my hands, especially during the COVID-19 pandemic, it was natural that I would dust off some of my best medical stories to further my understanding of 40 years in medicine.

Ever since I was a small boy, I've struggled with the concept of permanence. I'm sure it started after my father's death. And the concept of legacy has always puzzled and frightened me. For many, myself included, there is a strong wish to have something remain after life's completion. I guess, in part, it's ego gratification. But also, a desire that my future progeny will know something more about me than just a name attached to a faded picture on the wall. I hope these true stories, as told by my factitious elderly self, fulfil that aspiration.

Enjoy your travels back and forth from Providence, Rhode Island to Philadelphia, Iceland, New Mexico, Guatemala, Russia, Lesotho, Rwanda, Kenya, and Ethiopia, all important stops on my medical career path.

Barrington, Rhode Island
August 15, 2021

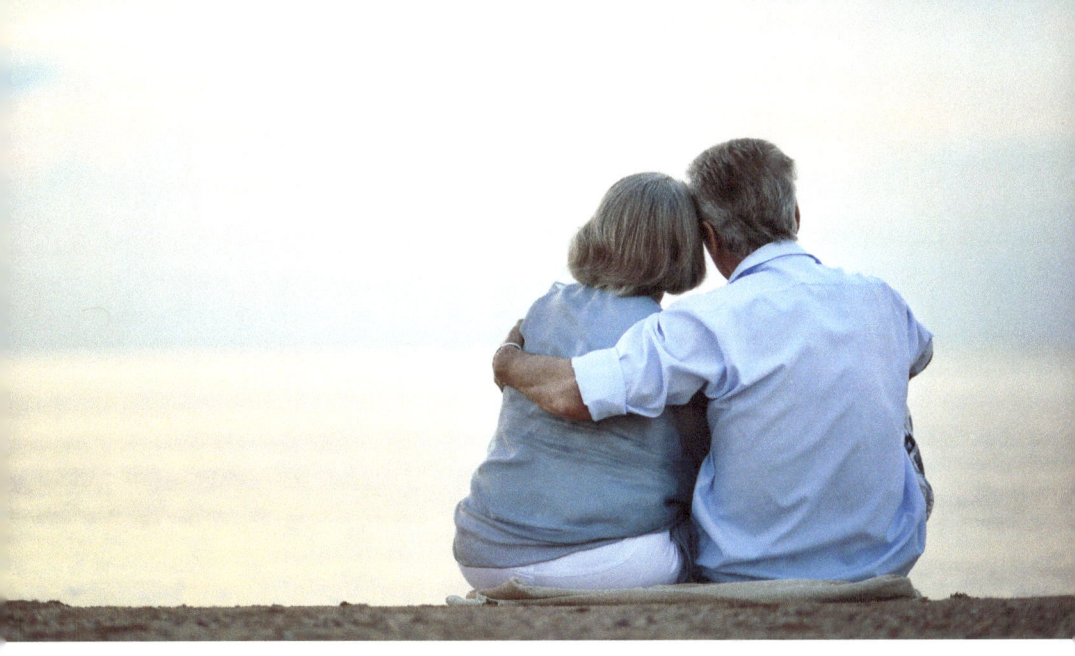

1

TAKE TWO ASPIRIN

"I'm worse, doctor."

"How can you be worse Mrs. Hughes? Last week you told me you were just about dead."

"I'm worse, doctor, and you just don't care."

How many times had we been down this pathway? Who else in their right mind would spend an hour every other week trying to help this elderly, intelligent, and "passive aggressive" patient?

Despite her diminutive stature, Mrs. Hughes possessed the force of a tsunami, one that could easily drown all in her reach. Even with the extra time allotted for the visit, I am close to running late again. I am trying hard to concentrate on her myriad of complaints, but her list is totally overwhelming me. I wish I could just prescribe two aspirin and send her on her way.

I momentarily drift away and realize in a month I will be back caring for patients in Addis Ababa, Ethiopia with its noisy pockmarked streets, luxury buildings juxtapositioned next to tin roofed shacks, solemn religious woman dressed all in white, and festive communal meals eaten with injera, the national spongy sour bread.

"Are you listening, doctor? You don't seem to be all here today."

I snap back to Mrs. Hughes, my exam room in Providence, Rhode Island, and the task at hand.

"Let's try to fix one problem today, shall we? Which one should we work on?"

"Oh doctor, I brought you a list of newspaper articles that may help. Can you look at them now?"

Is she kidding? I don't have that kind of time right now.

I take a quick look at the stack and say, "How about we stick to your heartburn today? This article lists foods you should avoid. What do you think about eliminating coffee for a week to see if that helps?"

"Oh doctor, how will that help? I'm so sick."

Mrs. Hughes has one of the most impressive whines of anyone I have ever known.

This really isn't working, I think to myself. These last six visits haven't helped either of us.

I close my computer and put the articles aside.

"Mrs. Hughes, how did you meet your husband?"

"What? Why do you want to know?"

"Just curious, dear."

Her face lights up. "Well, I was working at the Rhode Island State House, and he was a lobbyist."

And off she goes, taking me down the path of her early romance, wedding, and honeymoon. Her life with her husband of 45 years had been rich and fulfilling until his sudden death several years ago.

I end the visit by refilling her medications but tell her next time I want to know all about her own work at the State House.

"Oh, thank you doctor. I feel so much better. I know we are getting closer to finding the cause of my problems."

"Yes, I agree."

I remember thinking at the time that loneliness was such a terrible disease and one that often went undiagnosed in the elderly. That day, Mrs. Hughes taught me an invaluable lesson, one that served me well throughout the rest of my medical career. Sometimes the best cure for persistent and seemingly unrelated complaints is not more medications or more diagnostic testing, but just a few minutes of real personal attention.

"Dr. Charles, Dr. Charles. It's time for you to take your medication."

"Thanks Beth. I guess I was just reminiscing a bit."

I looked around our small room at 10 Star Premier Redundancy Assisted Living. So, this was where I would spend my golden years. As one of my patients used to say, "The only thing golden about this time of life is the color of my urine."

I guess it wasn't all that bad. I still had my mind, even if my body was failing. My kids were nearby and would visit on a more than regular basis. And my dear wife of 60 years, Kathie, was still with me, a true miracle not just because we had been able to age together but because she had stayed with me all these years. My son, Steve, once aptly captured this sentiment by describing Kathie as "my mother, who never deserved such a maniac of a husband." I was so fortunate to continue to enjoy her touch, her smile, and her positive attitude which often buffered my own disaster-driven mindset.

I did hate being on the sideline of life, not taking part in the action. How I missed travel, with its new sights, cultures, smells, and tastes. I never did make it to all the continents, unlike my daughter, Mya, who proudly emailed me from Antarctica claiming the family title of all six continents. I did miss being a physician with its privileged intimate relationships and the challenge of solving medical mysteries.

CHARLES B. SHERMAN, MD, MPH, DGM

My eyes gazed on the small bookshelf. Ninety-six years of life and all I kept were some photo albums, some journals, and my curriculum vitae from the Warren Alpert Medical School of Brown University. I remembered the day my son read the last version of my CV just before I retired. He handed it back to me, all 26 pages, and said, "So that's it, a lifetime of achievement, in one document that fits into one hand. Was it worth it?"

He didn't mean any disrespect. In fact, I knew he was quite proud of my accomplishments. I did feel uneasy at the time, pondering if it was worth all the time away from family, delayed gratification, life and death emotional intensity, and constant responsibility of caring for others.

But now, with the mellowness of age and more perspective, I realized that those CV listings were just place markers for so much more. Each line carried its own story, chapters really in a remarkable journey.

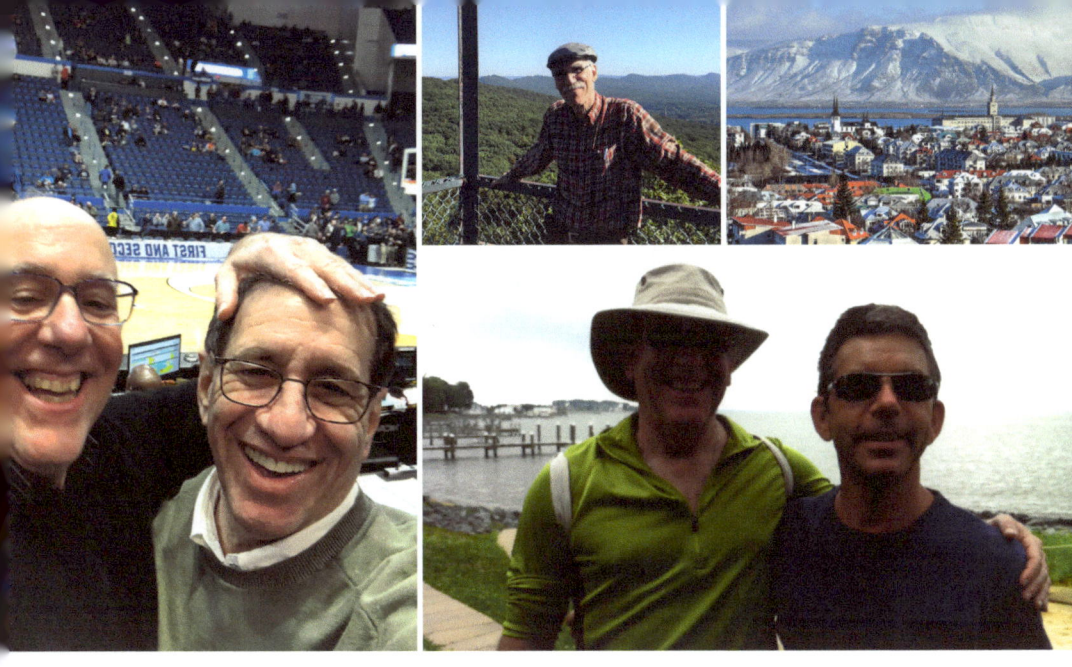

2

STAY RIGHT THERE

Mealtime at 10 Star Premier Redundancy Assisted Living was always interesting. I sat with the same people, just like in grade school where everyone assumed the same seat in class from day one.

My tablemates were Kathie and my lifelong good friends, Rick, Jeff and Steve, who had also ended up in the same facility. These were the people who knew me better than I knew myself.

Rick and I met in kindergarten and have been close buddies ever since. Rick is a kindhearted and creative man who is one of the few people with whom I can share early childhood memories. Only he and I can laugh about Miss Schwartz and the elementary school art room closet.

CHARLES B. SHERMAN, MD, MPH, DGM

I first met Jeff during our college days at Tufts University, located in Medford, Massachusetts, just outside of Boston. Jeff is a confident person who has always followed his own inner counsel. He has been a dedicated friend, even at times when I would drift away. Over the years, we have shared many unique adventures, including the time we decided to look for Katusha rockets on the Israel-Lebanon border, only to be chased away by Israeli tanks.

I befriended Steve on our very first day of medical school at Hahnemann University (now Drexel University School of Medicine); I can honestly say, if not for him, I doubt I would have made it through medical school. He continues to be a thoughtful and multi-talented writer, singer, songwriter, and medical educator. Our medical school "Darby Creek" talks, times when we could safely share our deepest feelings, helped me on my own path of self-discovery.

The guys were known as "The Availables" as they were all widowers and 3 of only 5 men at 10 Star. The 5th gentleman was Judge Donald, but no one liked him as he still bossed everyone around as though we were in his courtroom. He was married to Liz, who deserved the Presidential Medal of Freedom. I always chuckled at the name, "The Availables," as my friends were really only available for urinating sitting down. But they did like the attention and had t-shirts made up with the group name. I knew they were more than a little jealous that Kathie was still by my side.

After dinner one night, when we were all still sitting at the table, I launched into one of my stories. I knew they had heard them all by now, but either out of respect or forgetfulness, they let me continue.

"Remember the time I went to Iceland?" I asked in-between sips of coffee. I still loved hot coffee, a remnant dating back to my intern days when I needed the stimulant jolt to work thirty-six straight hours.

How insane to think a physician could make any reasonable

decisions with so little sleep. It was a macho mentality. I still recall the words of one of my mentors from residency training. "When I was an intern, we were on call every other night, not every third like your group. Our only regret was that we were missing half the cases by not being on call every night."

Total lunacy.

"I remember why you went to Iceland. Andrea, right?" Kathie said smiling as she got up to go to talk to one of her friends, Bonnie.

"Not again," croaked Rick.

"I know, I know, I was the reason you decided on Iceland," chimed in Jeff.

"I'd love to hear it again, Charlie," Steve sweetly responded. He and Kathie were always the ones I could count on for their patience with my excesses.

"As you may recall, I was to wed Andrea, bless her heart," as I spat three times.

"I never liked her," Rick and Jeff said in unison.

Steve, the retired pediatric psychiatrist, was kinder, "She had her moments."

I barely listened to their comments as I was already rewinding to the beginning of the story.

I had been living with Andrea for a year in a small apartment in Lansdowne, 6 miles southwest of Center City, Philadelphia. I was stuck at home that summer in the sweltering heat, without air conditioning, studying for Part 1 of the STEP exam, which I needed to pass to continue my third year of medical school training at Hahnemann University. Andrea had gone off to Tennessee to work in a rural clinic as one of the required clinical rotations for her Physician Assistant training program, also based at Hahnemann.

I was feeling exceptionally down when Andrea called.

"Yes, that's right, I don't want to come back and live with you unless we get married."

"Huh, are you proposing?"

"No, but you should if you want me back living with you!"

I was in a vulnerable state of mind. I was so conflicted about the relationship and marriage in general that I couldn't commit. But wanting her back for all the wrong reasons, feelings of abandonment (a theme in my life) and loneliness, I haltingly said, "Sure, let's get married."

"Wonderful, I accept your proposal. I should be home next week, and we can start planning the wedding."

"OK," shouted Rick (his hearing was even worse than mine), "get on with it!"

I quickly skipped over much of the engagement fiasco and fast forwarded several months to the part that Rick wanted to hear.

Andrea's mother had called asking how I wanted the final wedding invitations to read. The small wedding, in the planning stages for months, was scheduled in four weeks. That's when my "Commitment-induced Asthma" (a diagnosis I made years later after my pulmonary training) kicked into high gear. I couldn't breathe every time I thought about marrying Andrea. I awkwardly replied to her mother, "Let me call you right back."

I got off the phone and knew what I needed to do and should have done months before.

I mustered up my courage and walked into our small living room. "Andrea, I can't marry you now and I'm not sure if ever."

She immediately teared up in disbelief and called her parents. Her father asked to speak to me.

"What is this all about? I'm coming down to talk to you. Stay right there." He was a large man, a farmer from upstate New York. To say the least, I was totally intimidated by him.

"OK, I'll be here."

I immediately threw some clothing in a backpack and headed out the door. Not the most mature response, but my flight reflex was in overdrive.

I had six weeks off between clinical rotations, a schedule planned in advance to allow a wedding and a short honeymoon vacation. But where to go first? Jeff's house in Boston, of course. I caught a train at 30th Street Station and headed north with mixed emotion, relieved at not marrying Andrea but unmoored and adrift.

"Jeff, you were a great friend. You welcomed me in without any judgement."

We spent a few nights brainstorming my next moves. Clearly, I needed to travel, which had always afforded me time to think and more clearly reconnect with my feelings without the distractions of day-to-day life. And for someone who craved control, it was a way for me to relinquish that false constraint and trust the universe to direct my destiny,

"How are you feeling today?" Jeff asked as we were having breakfast.

"A little hung over from last night's drinking, but generally cold and depressed."

"Perfect," he responded, "I know just the place for you to go."

"And that is?"

"Iceland. I'm sure everyone there feels the same way you do—cold and depressed. You'll fit right in. After all, it's a relatively small island in the middle of nowhere, dark and wintry this time of year. Just the place for you to be right now."

Jeff was one of those people whose breadth of knowledge was vast and whose opinions, often strong, were always convincing.

So, with no hesitation, I booked a flight on Icelandic Airlines and arranged with my medical school advisor to do an independent study project on the healthcare system of Iceland. That way I wouldn't lose all my vacation time. My organizational skills were firing on at least 2 cylinders.

"How long are you planning to stay in Iceland?" asked the stern visa officer.

"4 weeks."

"Really, what's your purpose?"

I was so tired and without my usual conversational filters. I gave him the whole story, getting unhitched, the large father who wanted to kill me, and my need to be with depressed and lonely people.

"Whoa, whoa, let me see your study letter." Clearly the agent had no interest in my personal saga.

I showed him the letter and he reluctantly gave me a visitor's visa, good for 30 days, which seemed like the right amount of mourning time in Iceland.

I found a cab and headed to Reykjavik; the capital city nestled on the ocean in the southwest part of Iceland. On the drive from the airport, my first visual impressions were of unusually dimpled, brown landscape dotted with green parks, and then as we made our way towards the incredibly clean city center, stone houses, and small buildings all with red roofs. I came to later learn that Icelanders were more concerned about noise pollution than air pollution as most of their energy came from thermal pools beneath the Earth's surface. They would actually reroute airplanes landing in Reykjavik to minimize the sound of the jet engines.

I checked into the Salvation Army for a few days to get my bearings. I shared a room with a short, stout Norwegian fisherman who often came back to the room late at night, shouting in a drunken stupor. And there was the young, handsome Japanese man who had been traveling around the world for years learning different local cuisines.

"How long have you been in Reykjavik?" I asked him as I put away my few possessions in the small dresser in our crowded room.

"Six months," he responded in halting English.

I thought, *How long does it take to make small sandwiches with cream cheese, cucumber, and no bread crust?* but I just nodded.

During my early high school and college travel adventures, I always gravitated towards long-term travelers who had lots of stories to tell. They were often lost souls who were not rooted in any one place, true citizens of the world. My Japanese roommate was one of those long-term travelers with stories from all over the globe, mostly focused on food.

I spent the next four weeks traveling around the perimeter of the country, making medical connections along the way. It turned out that the healthcare system in Iceland was more interesting than I thought. There was a national health program that served the medical needs of all citizens at minimal cost through state-run hospitals and primary healthcare centers. You could see a specialist for a slightly higher fee, but one that was very affordable. No employment-linked and private health insurances, no costly prescriptions and no institutional discrimination on the basis of race as in the US healthcare system. Of course, that last goal of no racial bias was easily achieved in Iceland where it was known through DNA analysis that all Icelanders were descendants from just a few original settler families. The Genome Project had taken advantage of this singular lineage to begin to link specific diseases to specific genes, a major medical breakthrough.

The Icelandic single payor healthcare system afforded all citizens with at least basic health care. This sensible model was in sharp contrast to the one used in the United States during my medical career. Too often, I had cared for patients with far advanced disease and limited treatment options, all because they did not have the money to pay for earlier health services. It was so frustrating. Throughout my time as a clinician, I provided free care to my patients who were uninsured or underinsured, much to the chagrin of my office manager but in keeping with my philosophy that health care should always be a right and not a privilege.

All the Icelandic doctors, nurses, administrators, and patients I met on my trip were extremely responsive to my endless questions, warm and friendly folks who often invited me for a meal or to spend the night in their homes. They filled me with stories of Iceland, their Viking past and their fascination with alien spacecrafts. This last shared characteristic was explained to me by one physician who said, "What do you expect from a country in the middle of the Atlantic Ocean with an endless supply of alcohol?"

My hosts in Iceland took me to the southern coast to see puffins, those cute penguin-like birds that nest in the high cliffs. I spent hours in outdoor thermal natural pools with sulfur laden mist draped around me. I made a short trip to the interior to see the stark landscape that so resembled the moon that the NASA Apollo astronauts practiced their lunar exploration there. My favorite remembrances are of incredibly starry nights and daytime glimpses of several of the active volcanoes, one of which Eyjafjallajokull erupted many years later in 2010, forcing Kathie and me to spend several extra days in Paris as all flights back to the United States were cancelled. Nothing to do but enjoy more French cuisine and art, a true sacrifice that someone had to make.

I re-entered my Philadelphia life four weeks later to face my recent troubles. In an unexpected turn of events, Andrea had taken up with a new love interest. He was the one who met me at our apartment door, wearing my scrubs. My scrubs! Evidently, I was easily replaced. To make the situation even weirder, he was the brother of one of my medical school classmates, the same one who had previously asked me to father her child as her own older husband was unable due to a previous vasectomy. Spoiler alert, I didn't do it.

> "What, what was that?" Rick had suddenly awakened. "That's a story I want to hear. Forget this whole Iceland debacle."
> "Later, I'm almost done with this one. Where was I?"

Oh yes. Andrea was out shopping, so we didn't have "the talk". I gathered up my meager possessions and left. I headed to a house in Ardmore, the town next to Wynnewood where I had grown up.

> That's when I lived with you, Rick and Steve, in the house on Wellington Road. That was the place where the cockroaches challenged us to enter the kitchen every day, and where we

played whiffle ball in the living room. It was also the house where we were too cheap to keep the heat on during the winter months, and one time, all the pipes froze and burst, flooding the first floor. Anyway, to finish my story.

I wrote up my Icelandic health service notes for a paper that not only got me independent study credit but led to my first medical publication. I never regretted not marrying Andrea, especially after meeting and marrying Kathie. It really did all work out in the end, reinforcing my belief in the line by John Lennon and then repeated in the Best Exotic Marigold Hotel movie, "Everything will be alright in the end. If it's not alright, then it's not yet the end."

"That's all boys. Now go look available for the ladies."

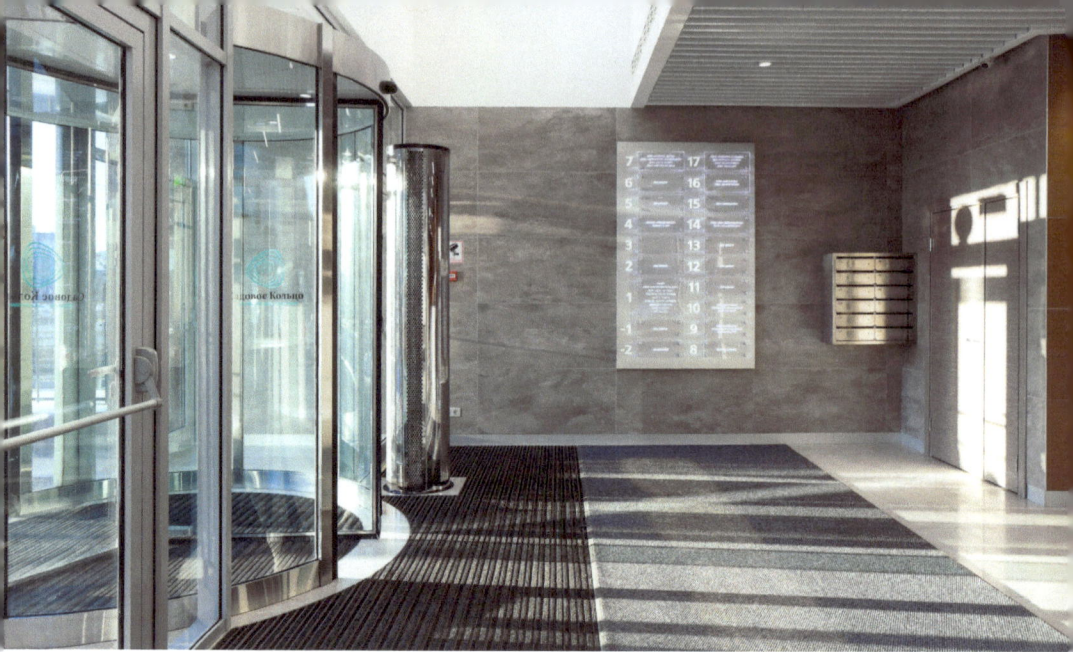

3

THE WORLD'S WORST HOSPITAL ORDERLY

Nico and Phoebe were our youngest grandchildren. They would try to coordinate their visits to 10 Star Premier Redundancy Assisted Living so they could see us and spend some cousin time together. Nico was in his second year of law school at Harvard where he was focusing on renewable energy law. He was hardworking, bright, and funny. Phoebe was at Penn, finishing her doctorate in artificial intelligence and specializing in the human-machine interface. She was energetic and charismatic. They were a joy to be around and shared a special bond being only 7 weeks apart in age.

"Truth be told, I wanted to be an astronaut or a photojournalist for *National Geographic*. But there was parental pressure, as in most Jewish homes, to have a physician in the family. My oldest brother Robert didn't do well with his science courses at the University of Wisconsin, so he bailed out and became a well-known artist and educator. My middle brother, Richard, applied to medical school but didn't get accepted. He went on to be a successful psychologist with a very rewarding career. So, it was up to me, the youngest son, to fulfill the family goal."

"One summer before my senior year in high school, I thought it would be a good idea to get some experience in medicine to test the career waters, so I signed up to work as a volunteer at a nearby hospital, Lankenau Medical Center in Wynnewood, PA. Remembering my first day still brings a little shudder to my soul."

I was assigned to the Emergency Department (ED), where my only responsibility was to transport patients from their cars to the entryway of the ED. I was so excited. I had my short white coat on with my brand-new name badge clipped onto the pocket. I already felt like a doctor. "Dr. Sherman," that sounded about right.

"Chuck, it looks like you got one," announced Glenn, the charge nurse. "Get the wheelchair and go out to that red Impala parked in the entrance circle."

"I'm on my way," I eagerly replied. As I approached the car, I thought how hard could it be to put someone in a wheelchair and bring them inside.

As I opened the passenger door, I said in my rehearsed doctorly voice, "Can I help you?" The patient was probably in her 40's, which was ancient to me, and appeared to be in pain.

"I think I may have broken my right ankle. I twisted it stepping off the curb."

"Well, let's get you inside to see the doctor."

I carefully positioned the wheelchair and helped her out of the car. I gently placed her right foot on the support. I pushed her up the short walkway right in front of the automatic ED doors.

I confidently pushed the button on the wall to open the doors. To my horror and the patient's, the doors opened out and not in and smashed into her injured ankle. Her loud cries drew the attention of the charge nurse who rushed outside and quickly took over.

When the commotion died down, Glenn thought it would be best if I did transport for another department like Radiology. I'm pretty sure she just wanted to get rid of me and possibly avoid present and future lawsuits.

My ego was a little bruised but still intact enough to allow me to make my way to Radiology.

Gianni, the coordinator in Radiology, greeted me with a sly smile. "I heard you had a little trouble in the ED. This should be an easier jig. Here, we pick up patients from the wards and bring them down for x-rays. I'll make sure your patients are healthy enough to get in and out of the wheelchair on their own."

This seemed like an even easier task, especially as I now knew that the automatic doors opened outward.

"There's a patient in one of the private rooms on the fifth floor that needs to go down for an x-ray. You good, Chuck?" Gianni asked.

"Absolutely."

I grabbed the wheelchair and eagerly sped off to the elevator. Riding up, I thought that the patient must be some sort of VIP since she was in a private room.

I reached her room, knocked on the door, and then slowly opened the door. The patient was an elderly white-haired woman in a drab blue hospital gown sitting by the side of her bed. She had 4 or 5 visitors, happily chatting with her.

I interrupted their conversation and explained my task.

The patient smiled at me in a kind way. I asked if she could transfer to the wheelchair without assistance. "No problem," she said.

I steadied the wheelchair and put an arm around her waist for added support.

Suddenly, she started to slip to the floor. I tried to grab her but ended up falling on top of her. Her family immediately started screaming at me, "Get off her, get off. She just had a heart attack and you're killing her!"

Somehow, I got both of us upright and her into the wheelchair.

I exited her room as fast as I could. In the elevator, she tried to reassure me. "Not your fault, son. I'm ok. I didn't realize how weak I'd become since being in the hospital. So, you want to be a doctor? That's nice."

In my head I was thinking, no way. Medicine is not for me. It's only been 2 hours and I've already injured one patient and fell on another after her recent heart attack.

Word traveled fast. Gianni was waiting for me in x-ray. His face was red, and his lips were puckered as if to blow me away.

"Are you kidding me? You couldn't just transfer the patient without falling all over her? And do you know who she is? She is the hospital president's mother, you idiot. You are out of here, go back to the volunteer office. I don't want to see you again."

I slowly and unsteadily made my way back to the volunteer office. Carole sat behind her desk and just shook her head.

"Wow, you really made a big stir around the hospital and in such a short time. Most student volunteers take much longer to screw things up. Where to put you, that is a big question?" She turned to face the window.

After a few minutes, she turned to face me and said, "I know just the place, physical therapy (PT). You won't have to do anything other than talk and listen to the patients. This should be a much better and safer fit for you."

And Carole was right. I spent the next several months in PT talking and listening to patients. We covered so many topics, families, careers, their injuries, really anything they wanted to discuss. I loved it. I also had free time to wander the hospital and watch other aspects of medical care. After that summer, as I went back to finish high school, I thought maybe being a doctor wasn't such a bad idea.

"That's amazing Saba. I think I would have walked out of the hospital right after the ER fiasco. I can't believe you and the hospital didn't get sued," Nico said as a budding lawyer. "I agree Saba, I would have packed it in right after falling on the patient. Good thing they have robots doing that sort of work now," Phoebe added.

"Well kids, it was a rough start, but I learned a valuable lesson that summer which stayed with me throughout my medical career. Listening to patients is really a key component of their healing process. Now let's go downstairs and get some ice cream."

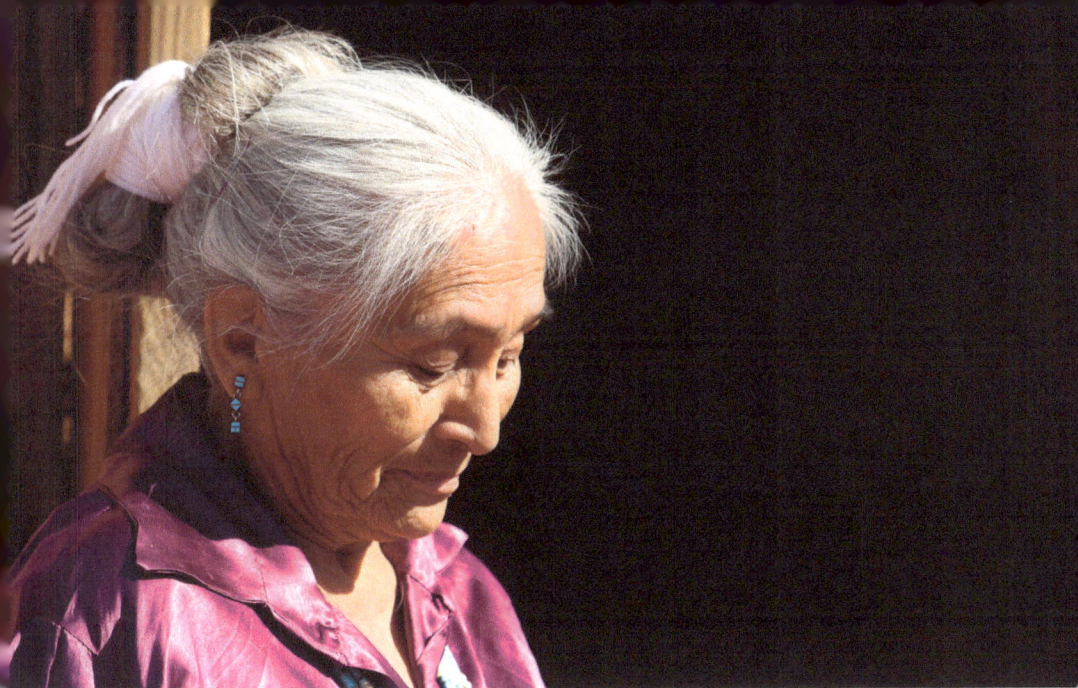

4

I CAN'T SEE

Early one morning, I picked up the yellowing copy of my professional curriculum vitae. Thumbing through the pages, my eyes first focused on the Postgraduate Education part.

1981-1984   Internship and Residency in Internal Medicine, University of New Mexico Hospitals, Albuquerque, NM

    I thought back to that first time I visited Albuquerque and the University of New Mexico Hospitals, and vivid memories flooded into my consciousness. If only I could as easily remember what I had for breakfast.

CHARLES B. SHERMAN, MD, MPH, DGM

I was in my fourth year of medical school at Hahnemann University and applying to Internal Medicine residencies programs on the East Coast. Several months before the application deadline, on a whim, I decided to apply for post-graduate training at the University of New Mexico (UNM) Medical School, located in Albuquerque, a city I didn't even known how to spell.

At the time of submitting the application, I was doing an elective clinical rotation at the University of Arizona Medical Center in Tucson, Arizona. I had picked that location because my high school friend, Dave, was living there. And when he had to go out of town for a wedding, I scheduled my residency interview in Albuquerque.

I flew Cochise Airlines, a small commuter airline that had a few routes in the Southwest. I knew I was in trouble when we were seated by weight and my luggage was stored in the wings.

We flew low over the desert at dusk. Dark green Socorro cacti peppered the brown shades of earth beneath the plane. A golden hue hugged the surface as the sun set.

We safely arrived in Albuquerque after the 60-minute flight. I waited in baggage claim for my luggage. And I waited and waited. Finally, I inquired and was told that my bags had gone on to Yuma, Arizona, the next stop on the route.

Panic ensued. I suddenly realized that I would not have my blue interview suit (the one and only suit I owned) until well past the time of my appointment. I also understood that I wouldn't have time to buy any new clothes. My nightmare continued as I appreciated that I would be trying to make my best impression wearing purple running shoes (with a fluorescent pink strip), blue jeans, and a polo shirt.

I went to the Cochise Airlines customer service desk to see what I could do to correct this most unfortunate situation. There I met a middle-aged, tightly wound customer service representative. She had a perfect smile which she knew how to use.

"So, can you get my luggage back tonight?" I politely asked.

"I can't do that, sir," she responded, smiling in a pleasant way.

"Can you arrange for my luggage to arrive before 8 AM tomorrow?"

"I can't do that, sir," she said, continuing to smile in a winning manner.

"Can you do anything for me then?"

"Of course. I can give you a toothbrush and toothpaste for the night," she replied, broadening her Cheshire cat smile.

"Can you do me one other favor? Can you stop smiling for a second?" I said in a less than pleasant tone.

"I can't do that, sir." By now, her smile was so large that her whole face seemed to disappear into glowing white teeth.

Muttering under my breath and stomping from the airport, I made my way by taxi to the Highway House on the old Route 66. I slept fitfully, worrying about my impression on the residence committee and concerned for my safety after watching a story on the local news listing Albuquerque as the murder capital of the United States.

The next morning, when I arrived for my appointment, all the other candidates were dressed in their finest suits and dresses. There I was, looking like I was on my way for a fast Sunday morning cinnamon roll at the Frontier Restaurant, a well-known UNM hangout.

To my utter amazement and relief, I saw that most of the attending physicians on the interview committee at the University Hospital were dressed like me, although some had substituted cowboy boots for sneakers. I found the faculty to be bright, interested in teaching, and very sympathetic to my plight. Many of the academic physicians had come from high powered East Coast programs, preferring the more relaxed atmosphere in New Mexico.

I returned to Philadelphia shortly thereafter and immediately changed my residency match list to rank the University of New Mexico Hospitals "Number 1." All of my medical school advisors told me I was "throwing away my career." I knew then, and I can reflect now, that training at the University of New Mexico was the right decision, one without any misgivings.

There were so many funny stories from my intern and resident days. The time when I asked my Spanish-speaking co-intern, Jorge Sedas, for help when I was examining an elderly Hispanic man.

"Ask him how he is feeling."

"Sure."

Jorge spoke very slowly and very loudly to the man, "HOW ARE YOU FEELING?" he asked in ENGLISH of course, just to see my reaction.

Then there was the time I was working alone in the Emergency Department (ED) late one night around Halloween. As part of my responsibilities, I had to not only take care of the patients coming to the ED but also field calls from outlying hospitals. I was tired and it was very late. I was on my own, which always made me anxious given my nascent skills.

The page came in overhead to pick up line 2. The physician caller said he had a real problem on his hands. A young boy had a carved pumpkin stuck upside down on his head and he was struggling to breath. No matter how much the physician tried, he couldn't twist the pumpkin off. He was worried that cutting the pumpkin would damage the child's face and smashing it could cause a concussion for the youngster. What should he do?

I had no clue. I blindly suggested he reach underneath the opening and spread olive oil and then twist. The calling physician put the phone down to try and voila, it worked. He thanked me and hung up; then the wave of laughter from the back hit me. The staff, including the ED attending physician, were all in the back listening in on this prank call. My initiation to the ED had been completed. They later told me that I should be thankful that I didn't get the scenario of the conjoined twins in cardiac arrest.

Another night on my "graveyard" ED shift, I was asked by the charge nurse to go outside to evaluate a patient still in the ambulance. I thought it was strange as the lights were off in the back of the ambulance, but as a dutiful intern, I went about my evaluation. I returned inside and told my supervising physician that I was certain of the diagnosis.

"What would that be, Dr. Sherman?"

"The patient is dead."

"Excellent clinical acumen, Dr. Sherman," as the room again filled with laughter.

These types of medical pranks were designed to lessen the intensity and stress of the work but would often seem cruel and unethical to non-medical people. I learned early on to carefully filter the stories for those of my friends not working in medicine.

My most poignant residency memories were from my time on the Navajo reservation, located on a wide swath of land in northern New Mexico. I spent 3 months in the town of Gallup, which was a rough and tumble place. Being on the border of the reservation meant that alcohol was available, explaining its raucous atmosphere. It was a common occurrence for pedestrians to be hit by cars on the sidewalks during weekend festivities. And it wasn't unusual to see patients in the intensive care unit (ICU) with alcohol overdoses, sometimes caused by the ingestion of Listerine or vanilla extract (both with high alcohol content).

It was normal at that time to see advanced disease on the Navajo reservation. Those living there often had limited access to primary care and a strong distrust of hospitals and Western medicine in general.

On hospital rounds one day, I saw an elderly Navajo woman with pneumonia. She spoke no English, only Dine, a complicated language spoken by the Navajo that was used in World War II to convey top secret messages. I explained to her daughter that her mother would be in the hospital for several days, receiving intravenous antibiotics, but I expected that she would make a full recovery.

True to my word, the patient did extremely well and was ready for discharge by day 3 of her hospitalization. On the night before her planned discharge, I was called urgently by the nurse to check on the patient.

"She says she can't see," stated the nurse.

"What do you mean?" I inquired.

"You'd better come and talk with her daughter."

I strolled into the room. The patient seemed fine to me. I examined her and again everything seemed in order. I told the daughter that her mother was fine and able to be discharged in the morning. I didn't know why she couldn't see.

"She can't see in this world because she has already crossed over to the next one," her daughter informed me.

"What?"

"She is transitioning and leaving this world. That's why she can't see."

I again reassured the daughter that everything was fine. Her mother's vital signs were normal, and her eye and lung exams had been unremarkable.

The daughter thanked me for my care, and I left.

Two hours later, I received a call from the same nurse who told me the patient had died.

I was and wasn't shocked. Medicine is part art and part science. But there is another dimension that is beyond our comprehension and often accounts for patient illness and recovery. My elderly Navajo patient helped me, early in my career, appreciate this spiritual realm.

One other vivid memory floated to the top as I remembered that story. The time I cared for a patient in the ICU who was terribly ill. I met with his family outside of the unit. I was used to having these physician-family discussions with three or four relatives. When I stepped outside, I was confronted with thirty sets of eyes.

One dignified gentleman took the lead and asked the important life and death questions. I informed the family that their elderly family member was critically ill, but we were doing everything we could. He politely nodded and then asked if a Navajo healer could see his father. I agreed, and shortly thereafter I found myself at the bedside with the shaman. It was surreal to visualize the ventilator delivering breaths, the monitors displaying second by second measurements, and the serene Navajo healer quietly chanting and swaying with his hand-held rattle. After a half hour, the shaman nodded to me and left. The family was very appreciative, which taught me another lifelong lesson, caring for the family is as important as caring for the patient.

Unfortunately, the patient died the next day. I was told that I needed to take the body immediately down to the morgue. My attending, Dr. Tempest (the quintessential internist who could perform upper endoscopy and also renal dialysis) told me that the family couldn't see the body.

"But they know that he died in the hospital, right?"

"Of course, but they can't see the body, or they will assume that his spirit is trapped in the hospital and none of his relatives will ever come back to the building."

Dr. Tempest reminded me that when someone died at home on the reservation, a hole was opened in the back of the hogan for the spirit to leave. If not, the spirit would haunt the family forever.

So off I went, pushing the gurney down the hallway. Suddenly, I caught a glimpse of some of the family members. I made a sudden turn and went down another corridor. But then, there were other family members coming that way. A quick U-turn and I was off on a different path, temporarily ducking into the stairway. Once the family passed, I ran with the gurney to the elevator and made it down to the basement without further encounters.

A spirit had been freed, and I felt like one of the Keystone Cops.

My time on the Navajo reservation set me on the path of a global health career. I had found caring for my Navajo patients so culturally interesting, medically challenging, and personally enriching. I was fortunate throughout my professional life to repeat this type of medical experience again and again.

"You know Nico and Phoebe, when I think back, it's truly amazing that I ever became a doctor".

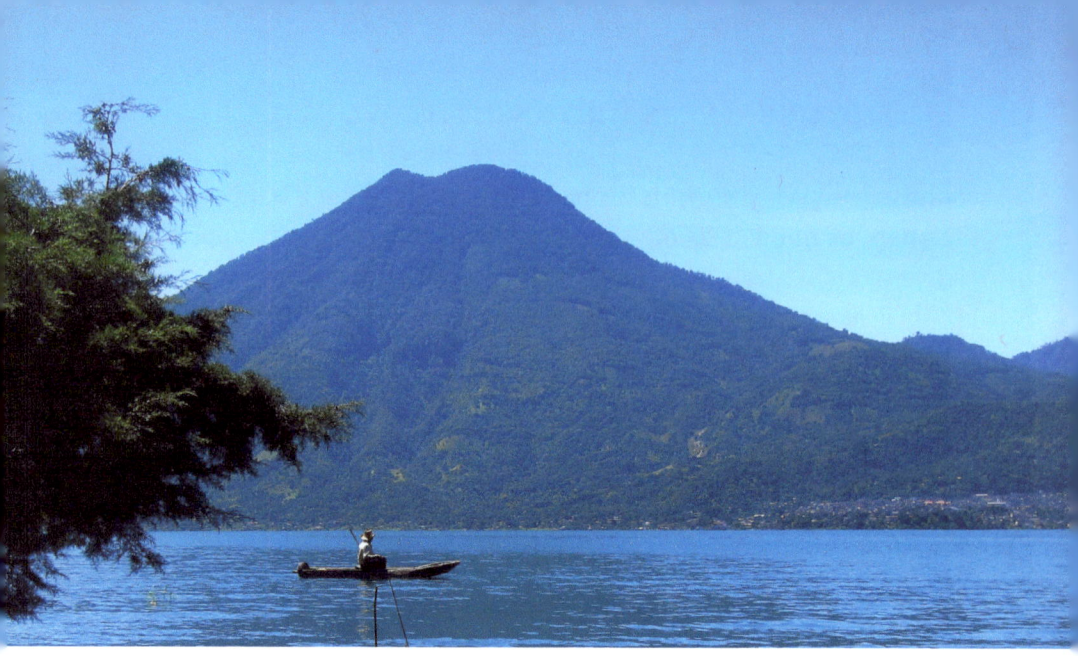

5

SMILE

Time in an assisted living facility, even a nice one like Ten Star Premier Redundancy, can still drag. Having Kathie and close friends with me certainly made the time more worthwhile, but I wasn't able to get outside as much as I'd like due to my severe arthritis. And there was only so much reading, talking, eating, and game playing I could do. Visits with family members were a treat but limited given everyone's busy schedules. So, I spent hours watching old television shows.

Through the magic of the Outernet, a more interactive and responsive Internet, I was able to access all my childhood favorites whenever I wanted. I loved watching *My Favorite Martian, Combat, The Flintstones, I Love Lucy, Leave It To Beaver,* and *I Dream of Jeannie.*

One afternoon, I was watching a TV show with my buddy, Rick. I'd known Rick for 90 years; he was my oldest childhood friend. We met in kindergarten and actually shared a cot during rest time. And I've never forgiven him for taking my graham cracker at snack time.

Rick and I had been through a lot together, especially during our early childhood. There was the time his pet monkey, yes, a pet rhesus monkey, got lose in his house, screeching and throwing things at us in his attempt to escape. The time we drank a pitcher of piña colada mix, stumbling up the stairs totally drunk, until we ran into his mother who told us there was no alcohol in the mix. Or the time when we bought a case of beer in bottles and a box of Saltine's and tried to hike 40 miles across Cape Breton in Nova Scotia. We both shared difficult childhoods and forged an unbreakable friendship bond to help us cope. In fact, we thought of ourselves as war buddies.

After the show finished, I turned to him and said, "That's nothing. Do you remember my story from Guatemala?"

"Who knows? I can't remember what we had for lunch. Tell me again. I always like how you stretch the truth to make a good story."

"It would be hard to make this up."

I was volunteering in San Lucas Tolimán, a small Mayan village on Lake Atitlán, an incredibly beautiful lake surrounded by three semi-active volcanoes in the western part of Guatemala. There were eight or so small villages surrounding the lake, San Juan, San Pedro, San Marcos, Santiago, and Santa Cruz to name a few, each with a Guatemalan health promoter (male *promotore* or female *promotora*) responsible for coordinating the health care of their villagers.

The building of the local healthcare system had been a joint effort between Guatemalan and US medical providers, under the guidance of the Mission of San Lucas Tolimán and Dr. Paul Wise from the Stanford University School of Medicine. The design was based on the sustainable concept of working within the existing organizational structure to improve the clinical skills of local *promotores* and *promotoras* and to obtain necessary medications and equipment from the Ministry of Public Health and Welfare of Guatemala. This model was unique at the time as most global health programs were based on the "duffle bag" perception of care. Well-meaning foreign health care workers, mostly Americans, would load large duffle bags full of medicines and set up short-term independent clinics in different areas of Guatemala to temporarily treat chronic medical conditions. This band aid approach rarely helped anyone and was one I could never really understand or support.

The medical work was just one part of the Mission of San Lucas Tolimán, which was started in the 1960's by Monsignor Gregory Thomas Schaffer from Minnesota. Over the years, hundreds of volunteers from the US worked with countless Guatemalans living around Lake Atitlán to improve education, economics, women's rights, as well as health care in the region.

My main task in Guatemala was to help increase early diagnosis and treatment of tuberculosis (TB) in the area given my background in lung diseases including TB. This was especially timely as it was predicted that HIV would soon overwhelm Guatemala, and it was well known that with a rapid spread of AIDS, a high incidence of pulmonary TB disease usually follows.

I worked with two other US health care providers, Dr. Bobby Gottleib and Nurse Practitioner Linda Foxworthy, both from Boston, on the TB project. The three of us would return to San Lucas Tolimán at least once a year, in two-week blocks, to help advance the work in collaboration with all the community elected health *promotores* and *promotoras* and the National Tuberculosis Program.

At first, we trained the local health care providers as cough monitors, collecting sputum on anyone in the village with a chronic cough of two weeks duration. The sputum specimens would then be brought to the regional government laboratory for analysis, looking for the rod-shaped mycobacterium that could indicate the presence of TB.

HOUSE CALLS AROUND THE WORLD

As the next step, we taught the health *promotores* and *promotoras* how to be direct observed therapy (DOT) coordinators, bringing medications to those diagnosed with TB each day to ensure adherence to the treatment program. One of the difficulties in treating patients with TB is the prolonged course of therapy, at least six months, which needs to be closely supervised to avoid the development of resistant strains of the bacteria.

As a group, we would go out early each morning to the surrounding villages, seated in the open bed of brightly decorated pickup trucks. These were safer than the other available public transportation, the chicken bus (*"camioneta de pollos"*), a modified North American school bus embellished with colored beads and crammed with passengers, animals (yes, chickens), and bundles of food from the market.

We were often joined in our pickup by men going to the local sugarcane *fincas* (farms) and mothers with their young children on their way to the larger market in Panajachel on the other side of the lake. Panajachel was often called "Panaja-gringo" for all the Americans that settled there, many to avoid the Vietnam War draft.

As we made our way to the villages, the air was clean, the sky was blue with puffy cotton ball clouds, and the landscape marked by lush green rolling hills in contrast to the tall brown volcanos, peeking out in all directions. Every once in a while, I'd get a glimpse of Lake Atitlán, its grandeur stretching out to the distant horizon.

> "Ricko, are you awake. I haven't even gotten to the good part yet."
>
> "You better hurry up; I might not be alive by the end of the story at this rate."

One day, instead of working on the TB project, we went to a school in Providencia to help with fluoride treatment of school children. My son and daughter were both with me on that Guatemala trip and accompanied Bobby, Linda, and me to the school.

Our task was to put fluoride paste onto plastic mouthpieces

that were then placed inside the mouths of the students for two minutes. The thought was that this would reduce the rate of cavities in the children as the community water did not have fluoride. The *promotore* or *promotora* for that village would also give the students information about dental care and send them home with a new toothbrush and toothpaste. This procedure was done twice a year for all grade school children in villages around the lake.

"Another example of well-meaning global health gone terribly wrong."

"What do you mean?" Ricko was paying attention, much to my surprise.

I explained to Rick that many years before, a group of dentists from Minnesota had visited the area and noticed all the extreme tooth decay, especially in the children. So, with all good intentions, they had decided that fluoride treatments would end the problem and devised a school plan for the *promotores* and *promotoras*. The dentists paid for the treatments and donated their time to train the health care workers. However, they didn't really get enough input from the local team; the mouthpieces didn't fit the small mouths of the kids, and tooth decay was in full force by the time the treatments were given.

And the real killer was that after the kids had their fluoride treatments, they would go across the street to buy really sugary snacks and sodas at the nearby *tiendas*.

"*Tiendas?*"

"Yes, Spanish for small stores. They lined the street right across from the school. Impressed with my Spanish?"

"No, not really." Ricko would never miss the chance of a little dig as close brothers are known to do.

Honestly, nor was I. I'd always struggled learning languages, and Spanish was no different. I would try all the available programs, Babbel, Duolingo, and Rosetta Stone. In fact, before that very trip, I had spent hours with Rosetta Stone. The problem with Rosetta Stone was that the expressions weren't very practical.

I became an expert at saying, "*Veo al payaso maquillarse.* I see the clown putting on makeup." In all my time in Guatemala, I only used that expression once, at a carnival in San Lucas Tolimán, much to the joy of Bobby and Linda.

I'm so glad that now there are nanochips that can easily be implanted into the language center of the brain and reprogramed with any language at any time. I wish I had that technology when I was younger. But I digress.

"Yes, you do and I'm slipping into my final coma."

During the morning session at the school, Steve got hungry and went across the street to a street food vendor. He decided to buy several choco-bananas, bananas dipped in chocolate and served on a stick. My concern was that the food was out in the hot sun for hours with flies everywhere. But Steve ate two before we could discuss the issue further.

"How were they?"

"Great"

We finished up at the school and found a pickup truck to take us back to San Lucas Tolimán.

That night, Steve started to get sick, vomiting, stomach cramps, and diarrhea. Fortunately, I had some World Health Organization (WHO) rehydration formula which helped keep his fluid status close to normal. By the next morning, he was feeling better. I still thought it best that he stay back and continue to recover from his ill-fated food adventure.

Mya, Bobby, Linda, and I headed out to San Juan to work with the local *promotore* to do more direct observed therapy work.

The day was uneventful. We worked with Vincente, who was one of the head *promotores*. He was a quiet man with an easy smile and incredibly smart. We had a list of all the patients that were currently on treatment in the village. Slowly, we made our rounds. At each house, Vincente asked how the patient was feeling, gave them the medications, and watched them swallow the pills. This practice of DOT had been proven time and time again to ensure TB disease cure.

Of course, it was never a short visit. We would enter the small houses, all made of adobe brick with a tin roof that would loudly echo during the rainy season. We would sit with the women and their many slightly shy children, eating *empanadas* and drinking *limonada con soda* (lemonade with sparkling bottled water). The woman wore brightly colored embroidered blouses called *huipils*, and long patterned skirts. We had to travel to the *fincas* to distribute the medications to the men working there.

Once we finished our DOT efforts for the day, we jumped onto the back of a crowded pickup truck and headed back to San Lucas Toliman. We briefly stopped at the Miracle Mile, where regardless of which direction you were going, the truck always slowly drifted forward when out of gear, hence the name.

As we approached the town, we noticed government soldiers manning a makeshift roadblock. This was a regular occurrence. The military would set up random checkpoints to catch cocaine drug smugglers and generally show the Mayan people who was in charge.

All the cars ahead of us were waved through, but when we were at the gate, more and more soldiers surrounded the truck. Everyone was shouting and brandishing their machine guns. One of the soldiers who appeared to be in charge came onto the back of the truck bellowing orders. Again, my understanding of Spanish was so limited, I turned to Bobby and Linda for an explanation. I became nervous when I saw the fear on their faces. I pulled Mya closer and tried to reassure her. We all knew the stories of the military killing innocent Mayans and at times foreign volunteers during the country's recent history. But this seemed different. The soldiers were taking everyone but us off the truck and letting the others walk into town.

More rapid shouting by the leader, a small mustached man in his late 20's, "*Pasaporte, pasaporte.*" ("Passport, passport.") He used his gun to move us together onto one side of the truck bed. "*¿Por qué están aquí? ¿De dónde son ustedes?*" ("Why are you here? Where are you from?") Then he moved us to the other side of the truck. Bobby and Linda struggled to get out their passports. I had left ours back in the guest house. More shouting, dogs barking, more soldiers, more guns, more chaos and panic.

Kathie's only instruction to me before leaving for Guatemala with our two kids was to make sure I brought them back safely. And I had a sinking feeling that wasn't going to happen. Steve was back in town, in my mind, possibly dying from dysentery. Mya and I were going to be imprisoned or worse, shot right there on the spot.

At the very height of the tension, there was a quiet pause and then all the soldiers shouted in unison, "*¡Sonreid, estáis en Cámara Sincera!*" ("Smile, you're on Candid Camera!") We were still so confused. Out from behind the roadblock came several camera men, the soldiers all put down their unloaded fake guns, and started laughing. The leader of the group slapped each of us on the back and offered Mya a small piece of candy.

Bobby, Linda, Mya, and I remained in shock for several hours. We told our fellow volunteers back at the Mission what had happened. They, too, couldn't believe our unfortunate experience. After much discussion, it was decided not to say anything to the authorities. Fortunately, Steve had fully recovered from this bout of Choco-banana distress, although he was forever known at the Mission as the "Choco-banana kid."

The episode of *Cámara Sincera* appeared on national television the following week. We became local celebrities, even having people request pictures with us. But to this day, I still remember the terror I experienced for that brief moment and recognize how many others, including those doing volunteer medical work, have unfortunately felt the same before experiencing a very un-Candid Camera outcome.

"Wow, that was a good one, Chuckie," Ricko said leaning closer to me. "That makes the Candid Camera rerun we just watched seem so silly. Let's go get dinner. All this listening has made me hungry."

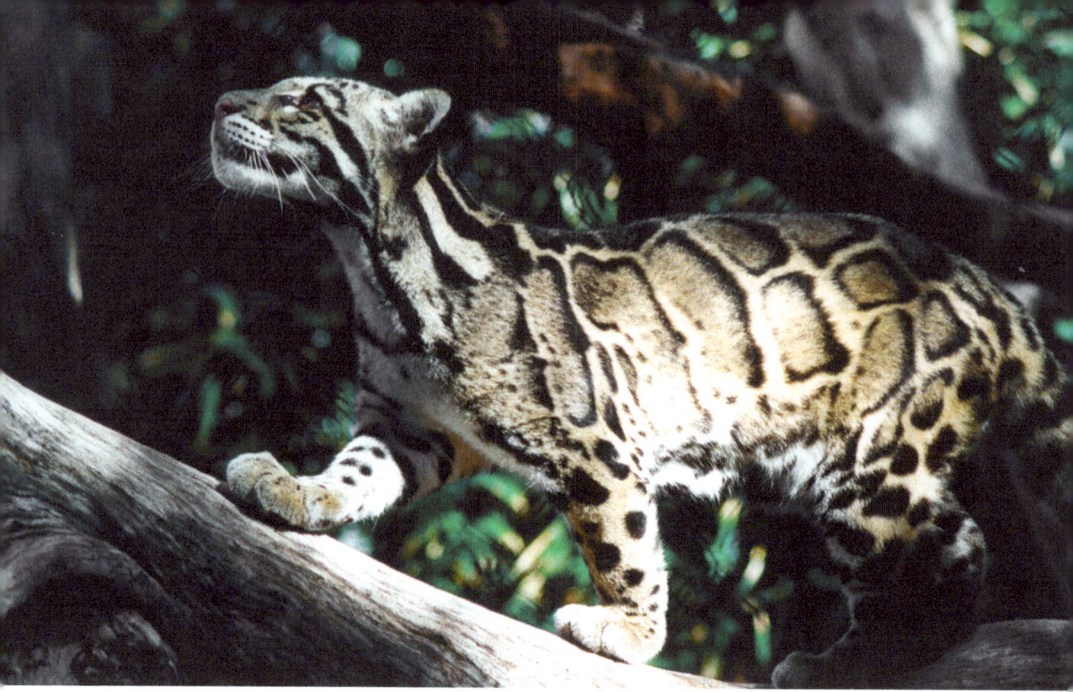

6

IT WAS A DARK AND STORMY NIGHT

I was gazing out the window in the sunroom when I saw a calico cat walk by the picnic table. It looped around two of the legs and then sprang onto the top. It circled a few times and then gracefully settled, facing the sun. Slowly it licked its paws and cleaned its face before drifting into a restful sleep.

Funny how my mind could so easily wander into the past. As I continued to look outside, I remembered that night at the zoo.

I was finishing up office hours on Thursday, seeing another of my worried well patients. My administrative assistant, Paula, interrupted saying I had an urgent call on the line.

"Hello, this is Doctor Sherman."

"Oh, thankfully you're still there. I need a big favor." It was Toba on the phone, one of my patients who also worked as a docent at the Roger Williams Park Zoo in Providence.

"One of the rare, clouded leopards has pneumonia and is getting sicker. Can you come and evaluate him?" There was a tremor in her voice. She loved animals, especially rare ones.

"Are you crazy? What do I know about pneumonia in leopards? Go talk to the head veterinarian."

"That's the problem. He's the one asking for help. He needs to know the organism causing the pneumonia so he can give the leopard the appropriate antibiotics. He wants you to perform a bronchoscopy (putting a small lighted tube into the airways) to get some specimens for bacterial culture. We don't have anyone here who can do the procedure."

A million problems immediately surfaced. How would I get a bronchoscope to the zoo? Where would we process the specimens? During my fellowship training, I had first learned bronchoscopic technique using a goat, but a clouded leopard, whose incisor to skull ratio was similar to that of a sabretooth tiger, no way.

But Toba was insistent. I finished up at the office and drove to the Miriam Hospital, where I managed to "borrow" one of the hospital bronchoscopes and grab some specimen containers and some microbiology laboratory forms.

I made a stop home on my way to the zoo. I wanted my family, Steve age 7, Mya age 5, and Kathie to witness this most unusual medical encounter.

It was a dark and stormy night as we drove up to the giant zebra painted doors located in the back of the zoo. The wind and rain swirled around us. As the huge doors slowly opened, I felt like I was entering Jurassic Park.

Toba met me on the other side of the doors, and we walked a few feet to the medical complex, where I met Dr. Jeromy Goodman, the zoo's lead veterinarian. He was a tall, classically handsome man in his mid 40's and very professional in demeanor.

"Hi, I'm Chuck Sherman, the pulmonologist all clouded leopards call when in need."

He barely smiled.

He briefly reviewed the case for me.

"The patient is a 3-year-old male clouded leopard who has been losing weight and lethargic for the past week," he said with a slight Southern drawl. He had grown up and done his veterinarian training in Alabama.

Dr. Goodman worried about an infection as the cause of his symptoms. He had managed to dart the cat with a sedative to obtain a chest x-ray two days ago. He handed me the film and sure enough there appeared to be a right lower lobe pneumonia.

The lungs of the leopard as they appeared on the x-ray were longer and narrower than those of my human patients. I made a mental note of how long the trachea, the main windpipe, appeared to be before branching into a series of smaller airways. I would need that information during the bronchoscopic examination.

Dr. Goodman then provided me with more information.

"I've given him several doses of Erythromycin, painfully darted each day, which is the appropriate treatment for a common pneumonia in a leopard. But he's no better and I'm worried."

Dr. Goodman's eyes started to light up as he began talking about the leopard.

"The clouded leopard is a rare cat. It is estimated that there are only 10,000 left in the world. It is a native of the dense forests at the foothills of the Himalayas, and has irregular spots and stripes forming a cloud pattern, hence the name. We've had our male for two years. He's always been healthy up until now. It would be tragic if we were to lose him."

Sadness and fear returned to his face.

I told him that I agreed that we needed to know the cause of the pneumonia and bronchoscopy seemed like the next logical diagnostic intervention.

"Can I meet my patient before the intervention?"

"Sure, right this way." He took me down a narrow corridor to a series of cages in the back area of the complex. My family had rejoined me to see the large cat.

> "Dr. Charles, Dr Charles. Are you awake? It's time for your lunch."
>
> It was one of my caretakers, Deborah. She was a woman in her mid-forties with an infectious laugh. She understood my humor and my love of salted hard pretzels, which she would smuggle into my room against doctor's orders.
>
> "Thanks. I'll meet the others in the dining area in just a minute."
>
> I drifted back to the zoo.

The clouded leopard was pacing in a small cage, looking agitated. He paused to stare at my young daughter for a moment, more to size her up for a meal than appreciate her sympathetic recognition of his discomfort. The cat was sleek and relatively small with a body of approximately 3-4 feet. His long tail whipped back and forth as he walked, quietly growling.

"Well, this should be interesting. How long until we can sedate him for the procedure?"

"Give me 30 minutes," Dr. Goodman responded. "Toba will show you to the operating theater."

Kathie took the kids to the aviary to watch the birds. I dressed in scrubs, grabbed the needed equipment, and followed Toba to the operating theater. It was a large room with a center table amidst a gallery of seats above. The room was packed with veterinarian students, zoo board members, and my colleagues who had made their way here for the show. One of my partners, Dr. Jim Myers, agreed to assist me during the bronchoscopy.

True to his word, Dr. Goodman arrived 30 minutes later with

the clouded leopard unconscious and breathing supplemental oxygen through a tube in his throat, an endotracheal tube to be precise. I watched as Dr. Goodman and his assistants positioned the animal on the table. Now that the cat was calm, I could appreciate his strength and beauty.

I sheepishly turned to Dr. Goodman and asked, "He's deeply sedated. right? He won't wake up during the procedure, right?"

"You're safe. Shall we begin?"

It was at that moment that I fully realized the enormity of my task. I needed to quickly examine the airways for any obstructions and obtain specimens so we could adjust antibiotic treatment, something I had done hundreds of times. But this was no ordinary patient, this was a rare exotic cat that was on the verge of extinction and could easily kill me if the sedation wore off.

We had set up the equipment in such a way that the viewing audience could watch the procedure on a big screen situated above my head. I was sure that my every move would be scrutinized by those in attendance.

Cautiously, I bent over, my face within six inches of the face of the clouded leopard and his large sharp teeth. His right paw rested above his head.

I carefully prepared to advance the bronchoscope into the endotracheal tube. Just as I was about to do so, Dr. Myers reached under the cat's paw and jerked it upward towards my face. Never being very good at handling surprises, I audibly gasped, which triggered a boisterous laugh from everyone in the audience.

"Well, I guess that broke the tension," I murmured to the group.

Using the eyepiece for vision, I guided the bronchoscope down through the endotracheal tube and the elongated trachea until I reached the carina, the sharp, main branch point for the airways of the right and left lungs. Carina is Latin for keel, the tapered underwater part of a sailboat. I first traveled down the left side, where the airways all looked normal. I then came back to the carina and preceded down the right side. At the bottom of the right lung, the bronchial tubes were irritated, reddened and swollen. I also saw thick grey secretions emanating from the distal airways. This was clearly the site of the pneumonia.

I washed the area with salt water (saline) and suctioned back the secretions for our microbiologic studies. I slowly pulled the bronchoscope out, getting one more view of the airways as I did so.

The clouded leopard did well during the procedure; his oxygen level remained above 94% saturation, a normal value.

I packed up the equipment and specimens and gathered the family to head back to the Miriam Hospital. I quietly placed the bronchoscope in the dirty utility room of the hospital's endoscopy unit for cleaning. I filled out the lab slips using a patient name of Matthew Leopard and submitted the specimens to the microbiology lab for analysis.

The next day I called Dr. Goodman.

"How's our patient?"

"A little worse for wear after the procedure. Any updates?"

I could tell he was really concerned.

"On the gram-stain of the bronchial wash, there appears to be a gram-negative organism that looks like Pseudomonas. We'll have the final culture results in a few days. Does Matthew (as he was now known to all) spend much time around stagnant water?"

"There is an area in his outdoor enclosure that is wet much of the time," Dr. Goodman acknowledged.

"I wonder if that's where he picked up the bacteria. Anyway, I'd switch antibiotics to a fluoroquinolone or a 3rd generation cephalosporin, whichever one can be given intramuscular via a dart."

"I'll ask around and start the new treatment today. Please call me as soon as the culture results are available." With that, Dr. Goodman ended the call.

The next several days passed quickly; my office hours were longer than usual with more patients as we were in the middle of influenza season. It was hard for me to understand why some of my patients refused their annual influenza vaccinations; I guess a misguided sense of personal freedom. Sometimes, I wished for a benevolent US dictator to mandate those necessary public health interventions like vaccinations.

On day four after the zoo trip, I got the final culture results back and sure enough Pseudomonas was the culprit. Fortunately, the organism was sensitive to the antibiotic the cat was now receiving.

I called Dr. Goodman with the results. He was grateful for the news.

"I thought that was what you were going to say. Matthew is already better on the new antibiotics. Come by and see for yourself."

After work, I returned to the zoo to check on my patient. He was back outside in his enclosure and looked like he had gained some weight. He didn't have that previously seen agitated appearance. Also, the area of stagnant water had been removed from his habitat.

I briefly saw Dr. Goodman. He was busy caring for a turtle that had a pneumonia.

"How can you tell?" I asked.

"They swim with half their shell up and the pneumonia side down in the water."

"Wow, how strange. Let me know if you need any more help in the future, although I'm not sure if bronchoscopy for a turtle is in my skill set."

He laughed. I knew then he was finally convinced that the clouded leopard would make it.

"Thanks again."

Dr. Goodman abruptly turned to care for the ill turtle.

I next heard from Dr. Goodman ten months later when he told me that Matthew had died from another pneumonia. He thought that the leopard may have had some immune deficiency which made him vulnerable to recurrent pneumonias. He again thanked me for my help.

Mathew was really not one of my patients, but his demise evoked the same intense self-examination as if he were. I went back over the case to make sure I hadn't missed any important details that could have altered the outcome. I discussed Mathew's care with my colleagues to see if they had any different diagnostic or therapeutic ideas. Finally, I tried to figure out the lessons learned from the case that could help me with other similar patients. This process was often time consuming. Thinking I may have made a mistake that resulted in harm to a patient was usually anxiety-provoking. But these additional efforts made me a better doctor, and when applied to non-medical difficult interactions, a better person.

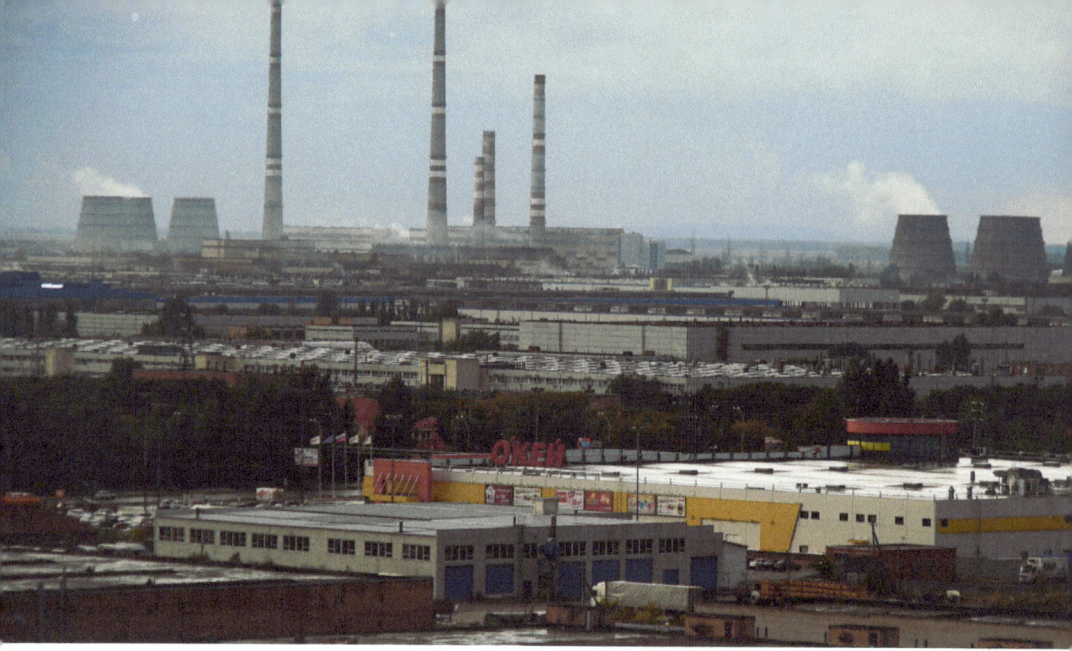

7

THE CIA PLOT

"Hey Yonas, can you mail a letter for me?"

Yonas was one of the new workers at Ten Star Premier Redundancy Assisted Living. He was originally from Ethiopia, where he had worked as a physician. He left his country in 2020 because of a civil war. When will humans learn?

Yonas couldn't continue his medical career without retraining, which at age 60 and with a large family, was impossible. I had first met Yonas when I was co-directing a training program in Ethiopia, and he was one of the first pulmonary and critical care Ethiopian trainees. He was an honorable man who was dedicated to his patients and his country. He would have been such an asset to any US medical team, if given the opportunity.

HOUSE CALLS AROUND THE WORLD

"Dr. Charles, how can I do that?" I thought that despite all his years in America he still had much to learn.

"Go down to the post office later this afternoon, ask for a stamp, and place the letter in one of the mailboxes."

"But Dr. Charles, no one writes letters anymore and there are no post offices. I guess we could use one of the transport drones to get your correspondence to its proper destination."

"Huh, I really am behind the times. Well, do whatever it takes to get this letter to my colleague and friend, Dr. Peter Karczmar."

"OK, Dr. Charles."

I had written Peter a long letter that morning. I had been watching a documentary about Chernobyl, a city in Ukraine that had been destroyed by a nuclear power plant explosion in 1986, caused, in part, by operator error. In typical Soviet fashion, the disaster was covered up and unfortunately led to the widespread release of toxic radiation throughout the world. The show helped me remember my time in Tolyatti, a small city in the southern part of Russia, approximately 1000 miles from Chernobyl.

Togliatti was famous for making the Lada, a small non-descript car that was widely driven throughout the former Soviet Union. The city was also known as the location of Stalin's summer home, on the Volga River, which ran through the center of town. Tolyatti was another one of those oppressive Soviet-style cities, tall gray buildings and concrete plazas devoid of color or nature, that were depressing even in the light of summer.

I had been asked to join a collaborative effort in 2006, The American International Health Alliance, because of my expertise in tuberculosis and AIDS. It was a time in Russia that TB and HIV were widespread, but the AIDS epidemic had not yet become apparent. The Russian government was masterful at total denial, "no TB and no HIV," despite mounting morbidity and mortality from both. My project responsibilities included assessing the needs of local physicians with respect

CHARLES B. SHERMAN, MD, MPH, DGM

to TB, TB-HIV, and opportunistic infections in HIV patients, and then developing a curriculum to address educational gaps through a series of lectures, chest radiology sessions, and case presentations.

Looking back, I started my medical career with the AIDS pandemic. I remember seeing my first AIDS patient in Albuquerque during the summer of 1981; a young man traveling back home from San Francisco who presented with a number of overwhelming infections, so unusual for someone of his age. No one knew at the time he had AIDS, that would take several more years to discover.

Interestingly, I ended my professional medical work with the Coronavirus (SARS-CoV-2) pandemic of 2020. I vividly recall my first COVID-19 patient, an elderly man who went from being a little short of breath with a small pneumonia to within hours requiring ICU level care for adult respiratory distress syndrome.

Both of these AIDS and COVID-19 patients died without a clue at the time as to the cause, a frustrating and humbling occurrence. Fortunately, in short order, dedicated scientists determined the responsible viruses and appropriate treatments for both diseases. The never-ending advance of medical knowledge was breathtaking to behold.

For the American International Health Alliance, I spent two weeks for two consecutive years in Tolyatti. And much to my dismay, just as our joint efforts were making progress to curb the AIDS epidemic and bring TB under better control, Vladimir Putin, the President of Russia at the time, decided no more American help. They would go it alone, and all joint US-Russian health care work would immediately cease. This was the beginning of another Cold War, which had previously ended on Christmas Day 1991 with the dissolution of the Soviet Union by then Soviet President Mikhail Gorbachev.

On one of my planned trips to Tolyatti, I asked my Coastal Medical partner, Dr. Karczmar, to accompany me. He was a logical pick as he was an excellent clinician educator and had grown up in Poland. He remembered having to sit through propaganda classes about the Soviet Union while in grade school in Warsaw.

I reread the letter once more before handing it back to Yonas.

Dear Peter,

I hope you and Cathy are well.

How goes the work at the vineyard? I keep waiting for my bottle of Beaujolais Nouveau from your grapes. Buying that vineyard in Southern France with your Coastal Medical buyout money was a brilliant decision on your part.

At Ten Star Premiere Redundancy (yes, I'm still here with nowhere else really to be) I was watching a documentary on Chernobyl which, in sharp contrast, brought back fond memories of our trip to Russia. I was hoping to relive some of those times with you, at least in letter form.

Do you remember those adventures in Moscow and Tolyatti?

I recall being jet lagged when we arrived in Moscow but dragging ourselves to the Bolshoi ballet where we saw Carmen performed. And then the next day touring Moscow with our beautiful young Russian guide, who told us in her somewhat stilted English that she was "young and flexible," which made us laugh. We visited the Pushkin State Museum of Fine Arts, Red Square (which was much smaller than I had imagined), Lenin's tomb where his body remained embalmed for all to see (he definitely looked very dead) and then that large outdoor market where I bought one of the original Sputnik satellite pins and you bought aviator glasses that you used on your moped for years.

I remember flying to Samara early the next morning and being greeted by Russian soldiers with Cossack fur hats and Kalashnikov AK-47 machine guns. It was right out of a Cold War documentary. Samara was and probably still is the production site of Russian missiles designed to carry nuclear warheads; it was strange to think that these same missiles were the ones with planned flight patterns directed at all the large Northeast cities where I and my extended family lived. In a picture taking mode, I snapped a few from the airport and was immediately surrounded by security. No one takes pictures in Samara, especially not an American, for fear of documenting state secrets of missile manufacturing. "No, we weren't in Kansas anymore," as Dorothy (Judy Garland) famously said in the Wizard of Oz movie.

We were met at the airport by our Russian counterparts and driven to Tolyatti. Our two-week schedule was packed with lectures, hospital tours, and ceremonial meals. I remember one such meal where I thought you were going to start an international scene when you accused the director of the hospital of taking blood money to work in Afghanistan as part of the Russian occupation of that country. I, on the other hand, just kept drinking vodka not knowing that I was supposed to wait for a toast each time before imbibing. Those toasts were long winded and always involved praise of the motherland.

Our two wonderful young female translators who accompanied us in Tolyatti not only translated our lectures from English to Russian but interpreted the culture and social interactions in real time.

"Talk to that person, avoid that one, don't say anything about Putin," and so on. I've always wanted someone like that here at home to help me figure out the motives and desires of those with whom I socially interact. The translators were state appointed and had some medical knowledge but not much.

I know I'm going on too long, Peter, and telling you things you probably remember yourself; I do enjoy retelling this story in great detail.

As you will also undoubtedly recall, our scariest time in Russia came during my last lecture to a distinguished group of physicians and scientists about HIV and lung disease, given in an ornate large social hall in Tolyatti.

"And it is important to always consider pneumocystis jirovecii in your differential when you find diffuse pulmonary infiltrates in an AIDS patient."

I then paused for the translator to relay my words to the audience. She went on and on and on. After she stopped, I asked her why so long.

"I really didn't like the way you stated the risk of pneumocystis, so I elaborated."

I never knew what she told the audience, but no one looked upset or confused.

At the end of the lecture, there was time for a question-and-answer period. Russians speak very loudly and animatedly when asking questions. At the beginning of my work in Russia, I thought the questioners were yelling at me until my translator informed me of the norm.

"Are there any questions?"

A stoic gentleman in the back of the room stood up and started yelling his question. When he stopped, I turned to the translator who had a troubled look on her face.

"He is telling everyone that the HIV epidemic in Russia is all part of a CIA plot. He wants you to comment."

Without missing a beat, I told her to translate my words exactly.

"That's funny because in the US, we heard it was a KGB plot."

The room fell silent. I thought, "Oh no, I did it again; I crossed the line and now I will end up in a gulag in Siberia."

After what seemed like an hour but really was only 5 or so seconds, the audience broke out in laugher, much to the chagrin of the person asking the original question. We left shortly thereafter for the airport, never to return to Russia. Too bad.

Anyway, thanks for indulging me.

CHARLES B. SHERMAN, MD, MPH, DGM

> *Do make sure to retell Cathy the story about when one of our other colleagues, Dr. Jody Rich, wanted to pay the prostitutes in our hotel lobby who were giving us information about the sexual spread of HIV in Tolyatti. He didn't want them to miss any revenue from potential customers during our interview time. That would have been a great newspaper headline, "US Researcher Uses National Institutes of Health Money for Prostitutes in Russia." Ha!*
>
> *Take care of yourself. I fondly think of you and Cathy often.*
>
> Best,
Chuck

I reread the letter with great pleasure as I relived my time in Russia. Before I passed the letter back to Yonas, one more memory floated back, our afternoon at the *banya* (sauna) in Tolyatti.

Saunas are an important social gathering spot for Russians. So as a group experience, Americans and Russians, we went to a nearby public *banya*. We donned wool hats and gloves and entered the dry heat of the wood paneled rooms, each wearing a bathing suit. We ate caviar and drank vodka, probably not the best thing to do in such a hot environment. I regaled my colleagues with stories of my previous *"schvitz"* (Yiddish for "sweat") experiences, first in Philadelphia and then in Boston.

As a medical student, I used to frequent a sauna in Philadelphia called Camac, named after the street of its location. The place had been around since the days of my grandfather. Men entered on the right while women entered on the left to segregated parts of the old gray building. I went religiously every Friday night for the first two years of medical school. Eric, my older brother Robert's childhood friend, and his father were my regular companions at Camac; we often had dinner afterwards. I always slept great after those evenings.

HOUSE CALLS AROUND THE WORLD

Camac was a throwback to a Jewish way of communal bathing, dating back to antiquity. Within the building, you could spend time in the swimming pool, dry or wet sauna, all in various forms of nakedness, draped in sheets. Or you could take a short nap in the chairs set up in the middle of the space. It was always a treat to see old Jewish men smoking cigars and talking business in the saunas.

My two favorite activities at Camac were the Turkish and Russian massages. The Turkish one consisted of hot towels draped all over one's body and a deep body scrub/massage done by a man whose breath smelled like a combination of cigarette smoke and wintergreen mints.

The Russian one was done in the dry sauna by men wearing large black jockstraps with their names embroidered, Moe, Henry, and Joe. They all wore sailor hats with hoses underneath bringing them cool water to allow them to stay in the sauna for hours.

You would lie on an uppermost wooden bench while the *Patchik*, the name of the person doing the massage, proceeded to give you a *Platza* (Yiddish for back or shoulders), which consisted of being beaten by a small broom usually made out of oak tree leaves and twigs, soaked in hot water to bring out the oils and aroma. Your skin would quickly turn a bright red, the concept being that more blood flow to the skin would detoxify the body. At the very end, you would sit on the side of the bench and a bucket of cold water would be poured over your head. As strange as it all sounds, the total body experience was exhilarating.

Much later, when I lived in Rhode Island, I found a similar though smaller *schvitz* in Chelsea, Massachusetts, just north of Boston. I would sit with my friends and the local Russians, getting platzas and eating lox and bagels on Sunday morning.

> I handed the letter to Yonas and watched as he placed it in the carrier space of the drone, which looked like a small jet.
> "Dr. Charles, I just programmed it for Dr. Peter's address in France. The drone will make several stops before reaching its final destination, but he should get the letter tomorrow."

CHARLES B. SHERMAN, MD, MPH, DGM

"Thanks, Yonas" I said as I shuffled back to my room.

On the way, I thought about how often political agendas interfere with better health care for the people, as exemplified by my Russian experience. How tragic that common sense public health measures were often thwarted by politicians, in the US and elsewhere, focused on holding power or advancing their own careers. This form of obstruction remained one of my professional frustrations, lingering throughout my career.

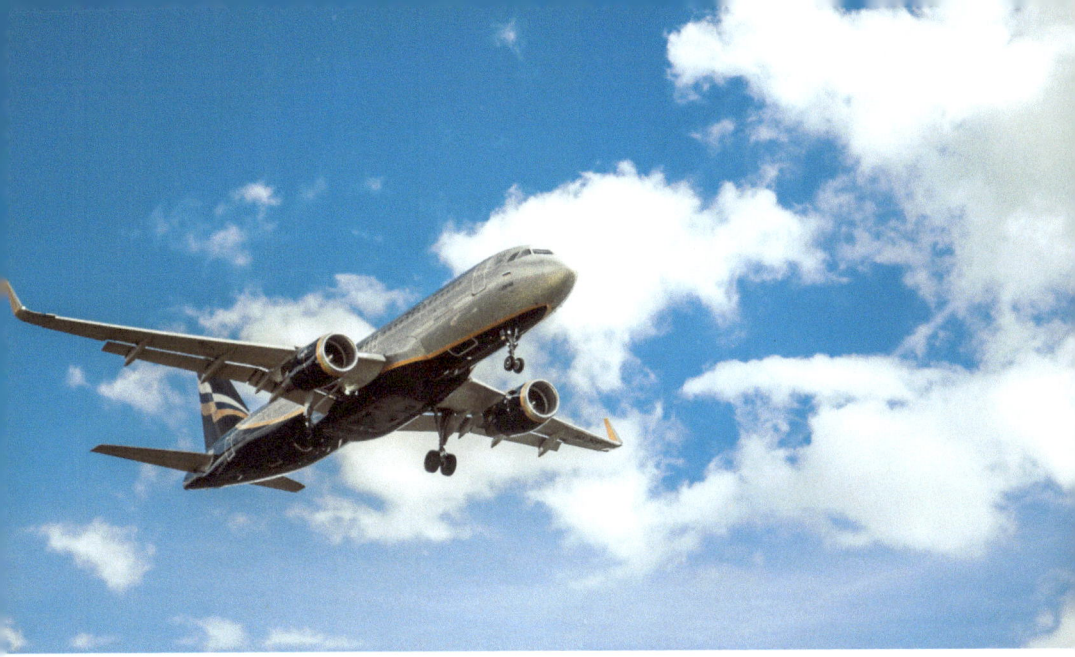

8
TO LEARN TO TRULY FLY

"Hi Saba. How's it going?"

It was my grandson, Rafi. He and his younger brother, Lev, are such wonderful grandsons; they contact me almost every week. Not on a cellphone, mind you, but on a system that Rafi helped design where his image appears as a hologram in front of me for a more meaningful interactive exchange.

I'm so grateful for their calls, especially knowing how busy they both are these days. Rafi has a growing family, my first great granddaughter Rachel, and an exciting career as a medical engineer. Lev just got engaged and is finishing a PhD in astrophysics. I just hope to live long enough to see some of their future accomplishments, which I know will be many.

"I'm still above ground. I haven't started peeing on the houseplants yet, and I'm not quite ready for my dirt nap."

"Oh, Saba."

After a few minutes of catching up, hearing about his wife's new position at the World Food Bank and learning that his baby was finally sleeping through the night (something my kids didn't do until they were much older), he reminded me about an important family observance.

"I'm calling today to remind you to light the Yahrzeit candle (the Jewish memorial candle) for your father, great grandfather Arnold."

"Wow, that time again. I must admit my days seem endless, but the years quickly roll on."

"Can you tell me again about that night? The night you found out about his passing."

"That was 87 years ago, *boychik*, such a distant memory."

"But didn't you record something 40 years ago for NPR's weekly segment called 'This I Believe'? I remember you shared the text with me when I had to do a project in high school on family stories."

He started to chuckle; a laugh reminiscent of mine.

"I also remember my dad's response when you first asked him if he had ever listened to that segment on NPR. I think his exact words were 'Oh, I hate those stories; everyone thinks their lives and their ideas are just so interesting.' And then you told him you had written a piece that you hoped he would edit. I love that story and the NPR one about your father."

"I think I have it around somewhere."

I commanded my voice-activated document program to find my essay entitled "To Truly Fly." And in seconds, the essay was displayed on my eyeglasses.

"Here it is, Rafi."

"Read it to me Saba."

"OK, here goes…

HOUSE CALLS AROUND THE WORLD

I believe that true personal closeness provides richness in life that is essential. I didn't always feel this way.

In 1963, when I was nine years old, my father was killed in a plane crash. He had gone to Puerto Rico with several of his closest friends to play golf. This was a first for him, leaving his family and going so far from home. He had never been a good flyer, often worrying that he would die in a crash. He stayed up late the night before he left, wandering the house and peeking in on his sleeping children.

On his way back home, his plane was struck by lightning and plunged to earth in a fiery mess. My family and I first found out about the crash by reading a news flash at the bottom of the TV screen during the Ed Sullivan Show. We didn't get full confirmation of his death until late in the evening, after I had already gone to sleep.

The next morning, I remember angrily thinking that life is unfair and unpredictable. I later resolved to do everything I could to avoid this level of pain and despair again, even if it meant lessening the pleasures in my life. I figured that if I never got really close to anyone again, I wouldn't feel so terrible when they were gone.

This served me well for many years. I graduated from high school, college, and medical school, maintaining an aloofness that didn't allow me great intimacy but also didn't cause me much personal sorrow. I was a solo pilot in the universe.

One night as a medical attending, I was alone with one of my patients who had myeloma, a cancer that ravishes the bone. He was experiencing constant pain; and despite all of our treatment, he was slowly dying. I asked him why he kept pushing so hard to hang on. He told me that these last months of his life had been the most meaningful. His family, previously estranged, had come together at his bedside to share fond memories and rekindle their love for one another. My patient witnessed with joy their new intimacy, and he felt that he could now let go.

CHARLES B. SHERMAN, MD, MPH, DGM

I pondered this man's sacrifice for many years. Gradually, I came to understand that death didn't have to be a dreaded event. I also came to realize that those deep ties between people, those moments of real personal connection, were the jewels of life. I was finally willing to drop my armor and allow closeness back into my life, regardless of the emotional price.

I write this essay on the 44th anniversary of my father's death. Over these many years, I have lived a rich life of intimacy in both my family life and in my work as a physician. In a strange way it was my father's death in a plane crash that afforded me the opportunity to learn how to truly fly."

We were both quiet for a moment.

"It's beautiful, Saba, a wonderful way to honor your father. You should read it every year on his yahrzeit."

"Yes," I replied overcome with a wave of sadness, "such a difficult lesson for me to learn."

"But one that you passed on to your family, for which Lev and I are so grateful."

We chatted for a few more minutes and then he had to go; I heard the baby crying in the background.

"Love ya, Saba."

"Love ya, Raferoo."

I deeply love my grandchildren, as I do all my family members. I guess I'm still truly flying after all these years.

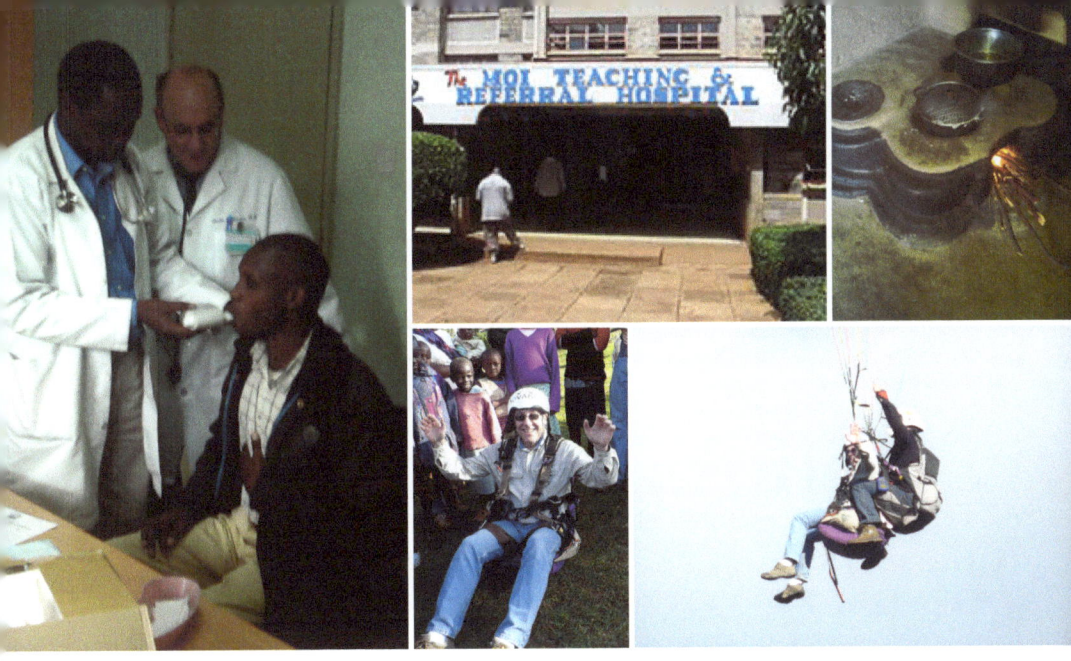

9

DIRECTOR OF GOOD MOMENTS

Diana, a diminutive woman with a broad smile came into my room with a container full of my daily medications.

"Really, I still need to take all of those? That's just ridiculous."

That expression was one my own mother, Ruth, used to say repeatedly. She was a complicated woman—smart, energetic, family-oriented, and judgmental. She made the best chocolate chip cookies and apple pies, never to be duplicated. She lived into her late 90's and taught generations of family members and friends how to overcome life's hardships.

"Of course, you need to take them every morning."

CHARLES B. SHERMAN, MD, MPH, DGM

"OK, I have a deal for you, I'll take all these pills right now if you sit for a moment to hear a story." Kathie had gotten up early to do chair yoga by the pond with her friends, Sue and Dori.

"I love your stories and you are in luck; I have a few moments."

And so, I launched into a story about Kenya.

I began with a little introduction to pique her interest.

I like the creative process of starting new activities and programs. The excitement in blazing a new trail has been an important part of my life. I started the naked quad run at my alma mater, Tufts University, with Doug Tase and other members of the lacrosse team. Who knew that it would take off and become a school sponsored event that my own daughter-in-law, Glenn, would participate in some 30 years later?

I began the New Year's Day Polar Bear Plunge at the Barrington Beach with my 8-year-old son, Steve, which was a strange one for me as I hate the cold, preferring to brush my teeth in tepid water. I kept annual records for years of the air and water temperatures and the conditions for the plunge—cold, cold, and sometimes colder. Over the years, so many people screamed and flailed as they dove into the icy waters for the annual ritual.

But one of my most important innovative efforts was bringing the Alpert Medical School of Brown University into the Academic Model Providing Access to Healthcare (AMPATH) program. Originally, this was a partnership between the Kenyan Government, Moi University School of Medicine (located in Eldoret, Kenya), and Indiana University (IU) School of Medicine.

AMPATH was based in Western Kenya and only consisted of a fledgling medical school (built by the Chinese, of course) when I first went there in the fall of 1996. Over the next several decades, AMPATH with the help of many, including myself and other Brown medical faculty members, grew into a multi-faceted health care system focused on the diagnosis and treatment of AIDS and tuberculosis, and then COVID-19 in 2020. And what started out as my first medical journey to Kenya blossomed into a huge medical exchange program for Brown medical students, residents, fellows, and faculty members. In fact, the exchange program became one of Brown's strongest recruitment tools for future medical trainees.

How this all came about still amazes me. In 1996, I was a pulmonary and critical care physician who was also a junior faculty member at Brown's School of Medicine. One lunchtime, I was sitting at my desk when I happened to glance at the ACP Observer, a journal I rarely read. In it, there was an advertisement from the IU group seeking volunteers for a medical exchange program at Moi University. I had always wanted to return to East Africa after my initial 3-month adventure to the area just before starting medical school.

I immediately called Dr. Bob Einterz, the co-director of the program. Within a few minutes of our conversation, he convinced me to go; surprisingly, the actual planning didn't take much longer. I walked down the hallway and approached one of the medical chief residents, Dr. Greg Kelly, who agreed to accompany me.

My first trip to Eldoret was energizing; I learned so much about diseases I had only read about such as Malaria, Dengue, Cholera, and African trypanosomiasis. I was fascinated by the cultural differences in medical care and by the skills needed to work in a low-resource setting. I knew then that I would spend the next part of my global health career dedicated to improving healthcare in Africa.

When I returned from Kenya, I shared my excitement with two other pulmonary colleagues, Dr. Jane Carter and Dr. Jim Myers, both of whom signed up for a month-long rotation. I also met with the Dean of the medical school who agreed to a bilateral memorandum of understanding between the medical schools of Moi University and Brown University. As they say, "the rest is history."

> "Dr. Charles, you know I have 10 other residents to see. Let me come back at the end of the day." Diana waved as she left the room.

But the genie was out of the bottle. I was back in Kenya.

Over the next 16 years, I made many trips to Kenya, teaching, caring for patients, and undertaking numerous research projects, mostly centered around lung disease and indoor air pollution from three rock cookstoves.

The tragedy of Kenyan patients dying because of a lack of access to health care, or a lack of resources haunted me for years. I could never make sense of patients dying from diseases such as asthma, heart failure, and pneumonia that were all easily treated in the US, often in the outpatient setting.

A series of pictures from the Kenyan wards quickly flooded my mind, two or three patients in a bed, far advanced disease states, and families serving as nursing staff responsible for feeding, bathing, and emotionally supporting their ill relatives. Compared to these patients, I had been taking care of the "worried well" in my practice in Rhode Island.

Superimposed on these many baseline challenges was the emergence of the AIDS epidemic, which decimated the region. If it had not been for the development and distribution of low-cost and "highly active anti-retroviral therapy (HAART)" treatment and the courageous efforts of a core group of US and Kenyan physicians, several more generations of Kenyans would have perished. But still, the number of patients I saw die each day was incomprehensible at times.

In contrast to this story of doom and dread, there was the optimistic, eager to learn Kenyan medical community. Making rounds usually meant traveling bed to bed with a team of 30 or 40 medical students, registrars (residents), attendings, nurses, nursing students, and pharmacists. All were attentive and thoughtful in their case presentations and questions. Their book knowledge was unsurpassed, but their ability to apply this up-to-date information to their resource poor setting never seemed to disturb them as much as it did me. They hung on to the belief that in the near future they would have everything they needed to properly care for their patients.

Diana kept her word and returned at the end of the day.

"I promise I won't bore you. I have two quick stories to relay."

"Do you mind if I sit and put my feet up. It has been a long day."

So, Diana and I both settled in. Kathie, who loved more of the activities at 10 Star than I did, was out playing bingo in the rec hall.

One lasting non-medical memory from that time was parasailing over the Rift Valley at Iten, a small community on the edge of a cliff overlooking an ever-expansive valley. This was the area where all the elite Kenyan runners went to train as the hills were high and the air thin, given the elevation.

The Rift Valley was incredible, stretching from Jordan in southwestern Asia southward through eastern Africa to Mozambique. The system was some 4,000 miles long and averaged 30-40 miles in width. It looked like a giant U with farms dotting the basement floor.

I had gone to Iten with a group of co-workers to have lunch, which of course included lots of local beer. The restaurant had an amazing view. Just as we were finishing our meal, a group of young men showed up to parasail. The steep walls of the Rift Valley provided the perfect updraft to keep the parasails aloft for hours. In fact, the record of 18 hours for parasailing was set at Iten.

"Hey, can you give my friend a ride?" shouted Jane, one of my colleagues, as we made our way from the restaurant.

An athletic young man from Germany quickly responded, "Sure, I'd like the company."

The next thing I knew I was strapped in, dangling from this huge winged flexible sail, with the German behind me, yelling instructions to keep my feet up after we jumped off the cliff.

Really?

We were going to jump off a cliff, tethered together with just a small bit of cloth keeping us from plunging to the ground?

And just like that we were flying. It was fabulous, riding the thermals up and down the valley. Every time we circled back towards the restaurant, I realized my friends were in greater danger standing so close to the edge of the cliff trying to get a photo of me.

After about 45 minutes, my bladder let me know it was time to land.

"I'm ready to go down."

"OK," said my German pilot, "We'll land in the cornfield below. Relax as we put down and keep your legs flexed."

Needless to say, the landing was not the gentle graceful event planned. We crashed through several rows of a cornfield. But in the end, all was OK.

It reminded me of parachuting with friends in college, when despite our training for landing, I basically drove myself into the earth at a higher speed than desired and came away with an ankle sprain, which was better than how others fared—a broken ankle, anxious times floating over high-tension wires, and a tree landing.

"And the other story, Dr. Charles?" I didn't know if Diana was bored or just wanted to leave for the day.

"Do you have time? I know it has been a long day."

"Yes, I want to hear the next one. Your stories are helping me relax before heading home to my frenetic family."

"I'll make it shorter all the same."

Our daughter Mya, Kathie, and I were on safari in Masai Mara in the southern part of Kenya. We were on a short vacation trip before returning home after another one of my two-week stints at Moi University.

We had gone out at dawn on a game run, driving around in an open jeep looking for giraffes, lions, rhinos, elephants, and cheetahs. It was a fun couple of hours, watching these animals engage in their morning activities.

We returned to the lodge around 10 AM and were sitting in chairs overlooking the savannah when one of the hotel staff came by to offer us food and drink.

"Would you like a beverage—juice, beer or other alcohol?"
"It's a bit early for alcohol, don't you think?"
"But it could be—you know—your good moment."
"Do you mean happy hour?"
"Yes, that's it, happy hour."

We declined the drinks, but I loved the expression, "your good moment." For years, I had been looking for a title for my work in Kenya. Visiting professor seemed too academic. Immediately after our visit to Masai Mara, I proudly took the title of the Director of Good Moments. And to this very day, when displaying my credentials, I put MD (Medical Doctor), MPH (Master of Public Health), and DGM (Director of Good Moments). Many of my old colleagues still refer to me as "DGM."

> "Thanks, Dr. Charles, for this good moment. I hope you'll share more stories in the future." Diana smiled and politely wished me a good night as she left my room.
>
> I settled back into my chair and for a lingering moment, I realized in many ways I had also been the DGM for my family and friends, a proud role to play.
>
> Kathie returned from Bingo, jingling her purse of winning coins. She gave me a kiss on the top of my head and awakened me back to my 10 Star existence.

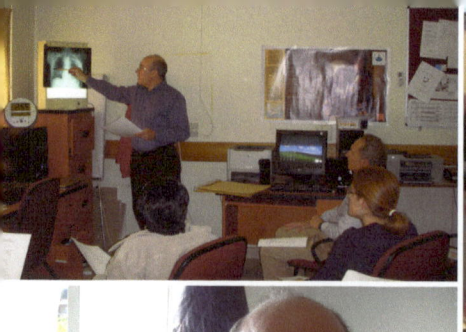
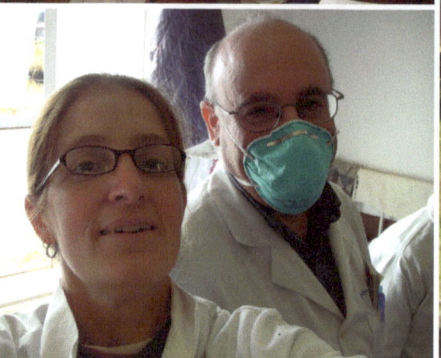
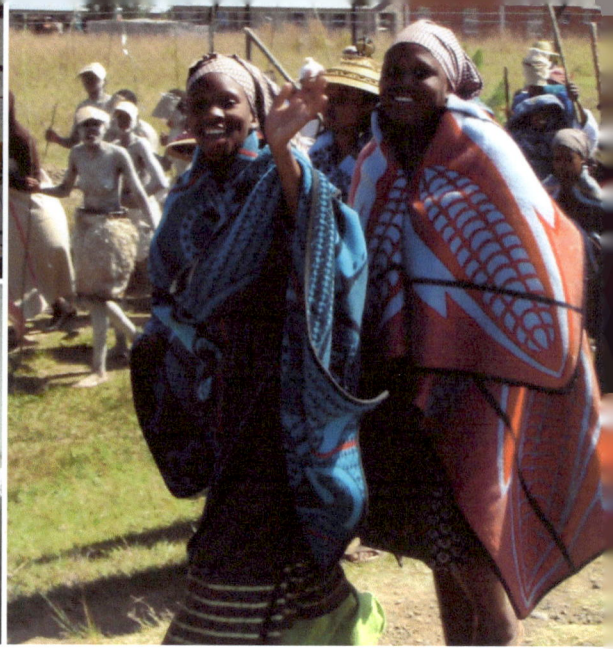

10

THE FLYING NUN

I loved teaching medicine. I did it for over 40 years, all across the globe. I taught medical students, interns, residents, fellows, attendings, nurse practitioners, pharmacists, and physician assistants. For me, teaching was part performance art and part scientific discussion of ideas. I gave lectures in traditional classrooms but also on sidewalks before Patriot's NFL football games and at restaurants before pharmaceutical sponsored meals.

So, when the activities director at 10 Star asked me to give a lecture on one of my medical adventures, I gladly accepted the invitation.

I decided to talk about my time caring for patients with extreme resistant tuberculosis (XDR TB) in Lesotho. I settled on a question-and-answer format rather than a formal lecture with slides as I knew my audience would immediately tune out and start dozing if I wasn't constantly engaging them.

"Where is Lesotho?" asked Karen, a frail brilliant woman who had been a bank executive. She loved to engage in philosophical discussions, during which she refused to tolerate inarticulate arguments.

Lesotho is a small African country, actually a kingdom, that is located within the borders of South Africa. It is only one of two countries completely encased by South Africa, the other being Swaziland. Lesotho is the only country in the world that is entirely above 4500 feet in elevation.

"What about the people, tell us about the people," shouted Penelope from the back of the room. She was a fairly famous writer of erotica. "It's not porn," she would always correct my friend, Jeff, when he made the accusation.

The people are called Basotho and the language they speak is Sesotho. They are a proud people who fought off many invaders including the Boers to maintain their independence. Of course, the British did colonize the country in the late 1800's. The Basotho men wear tall pointed colorful hats and wool blankets and often ride horses.

"How'd you end up there, Dr. Charles?" The question was raised by Liz, the wife of Judge Donald. As opposed to him, everyone loved Liz. Rick would flirt with her in front of the Judge just to get him to explode into a tirade of admonishments.
"That's a bit of a story."

I was constantly looking for teaching opportunities in Africa. A colleague at Boston University Medical School knew of my interests and forwarded a notice to me about a new Kellogg Foundation sponsored family medicine training program in Hlotse,

Lesotho. He thought that they could use someone with my skill set to teach for a short stint.

I had some time before my next scheduled trip to Kenya and thought it could be fun for Kathie and me to go to a different part of Africa. I contacted Dr. Fadya El Rayess, one of the core training program faculty members, and she thankfully extended an invitation for a two-week trip to Lesotho.

The trip itself was brutal, 16 hours of airtime, several connecting flights, a 2-hour drive to the hospital, and then an eight-hour time shift. Kathie and I were almost psychotic when we arrived in the doctor's lounge at the Motebang Hospital, just after the sun had set.

"I know you. I know all of you." I awkwardly spoke. Fadya, my program contact, was in the doctor's lounge at the hospital, but so were Deborah, her partner, their daughter, Alexis, and two younger sons, Anteneh and Abel.

"How amazing! Back in Rhode Island, for years, I have seen you all at the school bus stop on my commute to work at the Miriam Hospital. I guess I had to come half-way around the globe to meet you in person"

I love when worlds collide.

> "Well, that was boring," Rick mumbled.
> "That took forever to answer," Jeff chimed in.
> Liz in her consistently gracious manner spoke up. "Thank you for the answer to my question, Dr. Charles."
> "What was the work like?" chirped Jan, a spry, bridge playing golfer who was the local golf club champ. (The only other one in her age group was legally blind.)

I made daily clinical rounds in the XDR TB ward. Patients were critically ill with symptoms of chronic cough, weight loss, fatigue and night sweats. Unlike other cases of TB, the speed by which the bacteria caused systemic damage and the high number of medications required for treatment made this strain of TB deadly.

Of course, we had a shortage of appropriate medications, a

common frustration when working in low- and middle-income countries. I always thought that if African countries would pool all their resources, they could have a more than adequate healthcare system across the continent, but that wasn't happening any time soon. My main duties consisted of monitored the patients' XDR TB treatments and making suggestions to the local physicians, when appropriate.

TB has been around since antiquity. In fact, the granulomatous lesions associated with the disease have been found in the bones of Egyptian mummies. The disease is spread by air droplets, entering the lungs first before being transported throughout the body. This is why TB can affect not only the lungs but the brain (meninges), liver, kidneys, adrenal glands, skeletal bones, and the skin.

TB is more often a disease of the poor due to overcrowding and poor nutrition, and as you would expect those living in low- and middle-income countries are most susceptible. Fortunately, TB can be treated with medications, each with their own side effects, which need to be taken for many months, making adherence to treatment difficult at times. Patients with XDR TB present the greatest therapeutic challenges as most of the standard antibiotics don't work.

"I can go on if you'd like."

"No, that was helpful," replied Jan. "It's just ridiculous that the poor are subject to so much disease, both in this country and around the world. I read recently in the New York Times that with air travel so affordable, the global spread of infectious diseases is that much easier. So really, no one is safe until all are safe."

"You are absolutely right." Her last point was one of the important global health principles I had often taught to my trainees.

"Where did you live?" Judge Donald grumbled.

Kathie and I lived in a monastery run by a wonderful woman named Sister Lucy. She had a great way of saying "Yeeeessssss" in a drawn out slow Sesothian accent. She wore a long black habit and a white hat with broad wing-like extensions. The first thing Sister Lucy did when we arrived was to show us a photo of her flying, wearing that very hat, several inches above the ground during a windstorm.

"Like the Flying Nun," she laughed.

It was extremely cold and drafty in the monastery. Our fireplace was stoked with coal, which burned hot and dirty. We had individual heaters that we would carry to the showers to make the cold water less shocking. Holding my individual heater made me feel like one of the early NASA astronauts carrying their portable oxygen systems into their spacecraft.

Sister Lucy insisted on cooking for us each night. Her multicourse meals typically consisted of spinach and tangerine soup, maize porridge known as mealiepap (the national dish), meat or vegetable stew, and for dessert, special cinnamon rolls (makoenva). Those meals were a welcome treat after a long day in the hospital.

Any last questions before we serve our wine and cheese?" which I suspected was the real reason most of the audience was there.

"What fun activities did you do?" Kathy, one of the administrators, asked from the doorway.

We explored Johannesburg, South Africa, which was just over the border, hiked in the nearby snowcapped mountains, spent time at an incredible orphanage in Phelisanong, in the north of the country (Lesotho had lost a whole generation of parents due to AIDS), and visited a weaving center where women worked on large, detailed murals. One of those murals, a woman walking across the desert with her baby strapped to her back and a large woven grain pot on her head, hung in our house in Barrington, Rhode Island for decades.

"That's all for today. Next week I can talk about my experiences in Rwanda."

A low-pitched moan emanated from a part of the room where Rick and Jeff were seated. Good thing I was pretty much deaf.

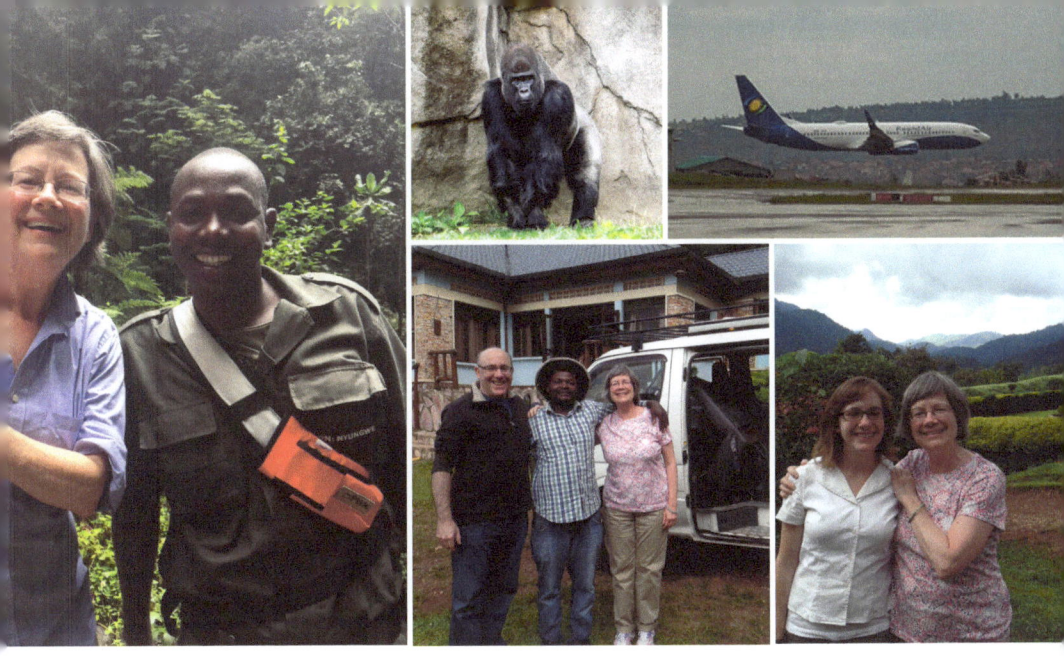

11

BUILDING THE RUNWAY

I brought very few belongings to 10 Star Premiere Redundancy Assisted Living when we relocated. I did bring a box of old travel journals, going back as far as a cross-country trip I took shortly after graduating from high school.

One afternoon, during a rainy day without much going on, I pulled out my journals and starting reading. I passed over the one from my 6-month trip to Western Europe, Egypt, Sudan, Kenya, Ethiopia and India, an adventure just before starting medical school, in favor of the journal from my time in Rwanda.

The journal cover was dusty, and the pages were starting to fade. But I quickly reentered a time long ago.

CHARLES B. SHERMAN, MD, MPH, DGM

MAY 5, 2015

Just arrived in Kigali for a two-month work assignment with the Human Resources for Health (HRH) project, a Clinton Foundation sponsored program. This is one of the few global health opportunities where I get paid a real US salary. I'll be in Kigali for a month at Centre Hospitalier Universitaire de Kigali (CHUK) and then in Butare for a month at Centre Hospitalier Universitaire de Butare (CHUB); both centers are university teaching hospitals.

Kigali seems to be a lively place, motorcycles buzzing everywhere amongst new buildings and well-appointed houses. After the genocide, money poured in from a number of high-income countries, guilt money really for their lack of intervention to end the killings. The money mostly went to build infrastructure, which is why Rwanda has some of the best roads in all of Africa. So hard to grasp the magnitude of the ethnic killings, some 800,000 people died in just 100 days in 1994. The current government has mandated the reunion of Tutsi and Hutu groups as if nothing ever happened. Talk of the genocide is outlawed. How incredibly difficult to forgive your neighbor when you know he was responsible for the death of your loved ones.

MAY 6, 2015

Orientation at the Ministry of Health. Discussed my role as a clinician educator. The HRH project is incredibly ambitious—training physicians, nurses, pharmacists, public health workers, and hospital administrators, all at once and over a short 5 years.

"We are building the runway as the plane is landing," explained the Deputy Minister of Health.

Sheepishly, I asked, "But doesn't that mean that the plane could crash before the runway is completed?"

"We have no other choice."

HOUSE CALLS AROUND THE WORLD

MAY 7, 2015

Kathie's birthday. We headed just over the border into Uganda to meet up with Mya. She's researching the effect of climate change and food insecurity on the Batwa, a tribe of indigenous people. Her research is supported by a grant from McGill University. We hired a driver on Mya's recommendation, which worked out great.

The customs officer at the border said he would let us into Uganda only if I guaranteed to make Kathie's birthday extra special. I promised and thought that spending time with our daughter in Uganda for Kathie's birthday easily met that demand.

We arrived at the Bwindi Impenetrable Forest in Southwest Uganda late in the afternoon. The area was lush with vegetation and jagged mountain peaks. It's one of the few primitive forests remaining. We had a fun birthday celebration for Kathie in the boarding house where Mya is staying.

The stars that night were brilliant, one of the best viewings I'd ever seen. The vast Milky Way spread out before my eyes.

MAY 9, 2015

Mya arranged for us to stay at one of the Eco-lodges, high on the side of a mountain, deep inside the forest. Our bedroom overlooks a range of steep jungle hills. The movement of the clouds over the peaks early in the morning was beautiful.

But the big adventure of the day was seeing the silverback mountain gorillas, who are the largest living primates and share 95-99% of our DNA. They are considered an endangered species.

We met our guide, a strong woman in her early 20's who was also a park ranger, and her two assistants at the base camp. It is never known exactly where the troop (family unit) of gorillas will be so scouts go out early in the morning to locate them. Some days, you do a short hike on level ground to find them; other times like ours you must hike for several hours, up sheer hillsides with the guides using machetes to clear a path. Kathie had a look of extreme dismay when she realized this wasn't going to be the short hike I had promised. In my defense, that's what had happened the day before. One assistant had a gun for our security, which added to the excitement.

After a strenuous two-hour climb, we finally met the troop, which consisted of one silverback male, several younger males, 4 or 5 females and one baby. We watched them for almost an hour at a distance of less than 20 feet. Of course, the baby was the cutest, full of curiosity.

What remarkable creatures. I'll never forget their bright eyes looking at us as we watched them. I imagined the dialog on both sides. "Who are these strange beings and why are they staring at us?"

At one point, the silverback male suddenly pounded his chest and made a run at one of the younger males. I really thought for a minute I was part of a King Kong movie scene.

Our trip down the mountain after seeing the gorillas was really one long slide. The rain, which had started, made the foliage quite slippery. The two assistants escorted Kathie down the steep slope. I couldn't tell if she was pissed at me or enjoying the escort service.

A truly remarkable once in a lifetime experience.

Mya seems well and enjoys her work. Great to spend time with her.

MAY 20, 2015

Ruth is back in the hospital, probably heart failure. It's a difficult situation as none of us are living close to our mother in Florida and my brothers are relying on me from afar to manage the situation. Thank god for Zoom and What's App, which have allowed daily calls to Ruth and her doctors. We really need to come up with a better living arrangement for her, especially if she continues to make frequent trips to the hospital.

MAY 25, 2015

Work has been stressful. I am spending too much time trying to fit in. The US internists who are working in Rwanda for a year are well trained and not used to having a sub-specialist around. I'm trying to find my way but it hasn't been easy. The overall program organization is somewhat chaotic. Let's hope that plane can land as they build the runway.

MAY 30, 2015

Leave for Butare later today. Looking forward to working in a more remote area of the country. We will be living with a US pediatrician, which will be a nice change from the rather isolated house where we have stayed in Kigali.

JUNE 5, 2015

Wow, what an improvement. The hospital sits on a plateau overlooking acres and acres of fertile farmland. The staff at the hospital welcomed me with a warm embrace. I've already started a lecture series and ultrasound training sessions. I finally feel like I'm making a difference. That's the trouble with these short global health teaching assignments, you never really know the need until you arrive.

JUNE 20, 2015

I haven't written in a while. The work here is everything I had envisioned. The medical students and residents are totally engaged, and I have started to make plans to bring the East African Training Initiative, our pulmonary and critical care training program based in Ethiopia, to Rwanda. Kathie and I have enjoyed the community of visiting faculty. And Kathie is quite famous in our neighborhood as the debate coach for the local school. Often at night when we walk, several of the school children will greet her with great enthusiasm, wanting to hug her. My favorite of the current debate topics is "What is more important money or friends?," a discussion worthy of us all.

CHARLES B. SHERMAN, MD, MPH, DGM

JUNE 30, 2015

Last day in Rwanda. Kathie and I are staying at the Hotel des Mille Collines (the hotel of a 1000 hills) in Kigali before we leave for the US in the morning. The hotel became famous for the 1,268 Tutsi people saved from the Hutu soldiers during the genocide by the brave hotel manager, who himself was a Hutu; all were safely hidden within the hotel rooms. I had seen the movie, *Hotel Rwanda,* before coming to the country. The hotel basically looks the same as it did then. I could just imagine the UN troops in the front of the hotel, refusing to get involved in the conflict.

My time in Rwanda has been one of the most significant in my global health work. And I think Kathie found her work equally rewarding.

I put the journal down and briefly reflected on the experience in Rwanda. I had made a difference in the education of many; just as important, I had shared with them a meaningful moment in time. A moment that allowed a cross cultural acknowledgement of the universal need for laughter, love, and the recognition of the value of others.

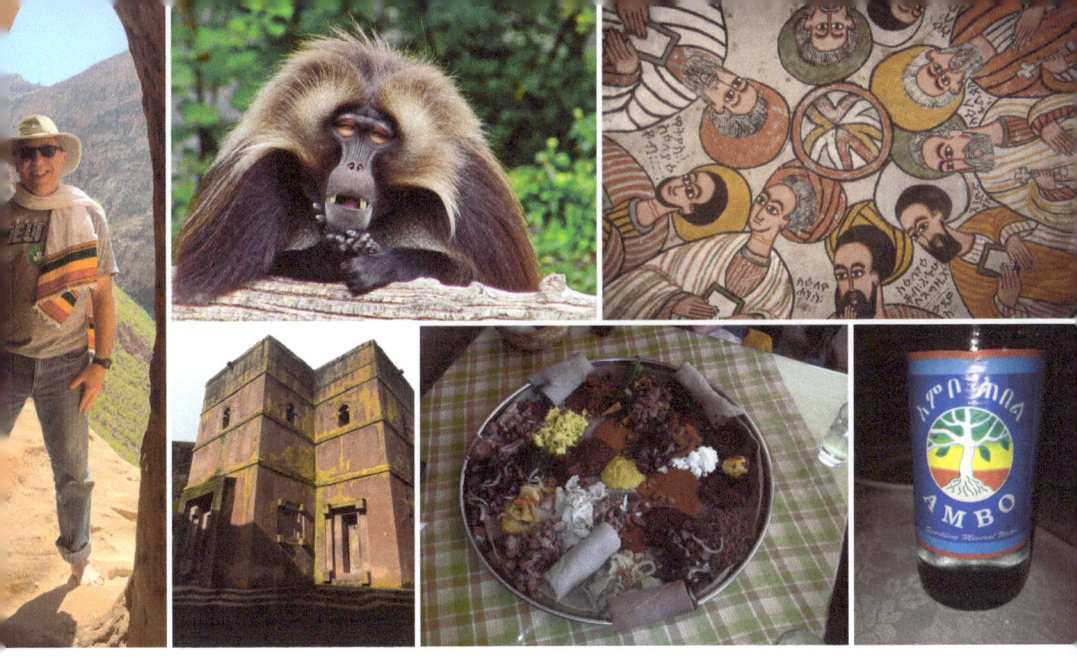

12

YOU WANT ME TO DO WHAT?

One day, Debi came to visit Kathie and me. It had been quite some time since we had last seen her. She was one of my closest colleagues when we worked together for the East African Training Initiative (EATI).

EATI was probably my most successful program, likely benefiting from all my previous years of global medicine. It was a 10-year project that trained 25 Ethiopian pulmonary and critical care medicine (PCCM) physicians. Not bad given that we had started with only 1 partially trained PCCM doc upon our arrival in Addis Ababa early in 2013. It was also my last significant project in Africa.

"How are you, Debi? You look marvelous." Debi was now in her 60's, which seemed amazing to me as I had first met her when she was in her mid 30's.

"Not bad, not bad," answered Debi, in her warm and friendly manner.

"What brings you to the illustrious 10 Star Premiere Redundancy Assisted Living facility?" inquired Kathie.

"I'm writing a book about the early years of EATI and wanted to get some more information from you both. After all, you were the first to go when the training program began."

The EATI program had grown so much in the ensuing years since the start that my own involvement was gradually disappearing from the collective memory. EATI was now totally self-sufficient with robust clinical training, research, and public health components. It continued to set the standard for physician education and health care delivery, not just in Ethiopia but throughout East Africa.

The rapid upward trajectory for the program's acknowledged success was, in part, precipitated by the COVID-19 pandemic of 2020-2021. During those years, the Ethiopian physicians, who had been trained by EATI, took on major leadership roles to help curb the widespread destruction of the coronavirus. Those many dedicated PCCM physicians were recognized by the Ministry of Health for their contributions, receiving numerous service awards from the government.

"How much time do you have?" I asked. "You may be here for a while."

"Certainly, the afternoon for starters." Debi hadn't lost her melodic verbal tone. "How about starting with the time you insulted the entire country, Chuck?"

"This happened years before you joined EATI."

I was giving Grand Rounds for the Department of Medicine at Tikur Anbessa Specialized Hospital, the main teaching hospital for EATI, on interstitial lung disease. Several days before the talk, Tola, one of the first trainees, had mentioned at lunch that injera, the national spongy, tangy flat bread eaten with each meal, looked a lot like the pathologic pattern of usual interstitial lung disease

(UIP) on one side with its honeycombing and non-specific interstitial lung disease (NSIP) on the other flat surfaced side.

During my Grand Rounds lecture, I showed a picture of injera and told the audience they should always think of UIP and NSIP when eating injera. I finished the talk and asked for questions.

One of the senior Ethiopian physicians, actually the first woman in the Department of Medicine, stood up and stated emphatically that I had insulted the entire country by my analogy. She insisted that I apologize and never mention interstitial lung disease and injera in the same sentence ever again. She could be extremely commanding. I quickly "fell on my sword" and told the audience I never meant to insult the Ethiopian culture.

For the next several years, each time we met, that attending physician would ask me if I had mentioned injera in any of my talks. True to my word, I never did again. It had been a humbling experience. Once again, the critical need for heightened cultural awareness when medically working overseas had escape my consciousness.

> Debi immediately said, "Yes, I know many at the time thought the program was a 'goner' after that lecture. What other stories from that first year come to mind?"

There are so many, several about other cultural differences I had to learn early on. Like the day on rounds when the intern handed me the most recent chest x-ray, and I questioned him about giving me a film from 7 years ago. The unfazed young doctor patiently told me that the date was recorded using the Ethiopian calendar which had 13 months in a year, 12 of which had 30 days and the last month had five days or six days in a leap year. So, in fact, he had given me the most recent chest x-ray just with the Ethiopian calendar date.

Or when I told the rounding team, we would meet at 7AM and no one showed up until 1 PM as they thought I meant Ethiopian time, which is based on two twelve-hour cycles with 7 AM considered the first hour of the day and 7 PM the first hour of the night.

Another learning experience was that khat, a stimulant, was something I shouldn't ingest. Taking khat is a custom among Muslims from the southern part of the country. You chew the leaves and drink coffee after a special meal, like Eid at the end of Ramadan. After celebrating one Eid with Fahmi, the other first trainee, and his family, I think I was up for 72 straight hours. No more khat for me.

My clinical time was often challenging. I constantly struggled with the lack of resources which not only affected patient care but infiltrated the mindset of the physicians. They were so used to not having what they needed to properly care for patients that they lost the urge to fight and demand for more. That was a hard, but understandable, perspective to change, but we did make some progress over time.

> Debi wanted to engage Kathie in the discussion. "Kathie, any fond memories of the Molla Hotel?"
> "Ah, the Molla Hotel," Kathie smiled in loving remembrance.

Chuck and I spent 6 weeks at the Molla that first year. The place was owned by Mr. Molla, a lawyer who had spent time in prison for political crimes, and his younger wife Gigi. We always thought the hotel must have been a tax shelter for them. It was a small hotel with only 12 rooms, all of which came with a stationary bicycle which was more appropriate for drying clothing than exercising.

The staff was great, always trying to correct any problems that arose; but despite their best efforts, the showers were usually cold, the internet didn't work most days, and the smoke from the ground level bar often drifted upward through the floorboards into our second-floor room.

Breakfast was always an adventure. Each morning Chuck would order an omelet and scrambled eggs would come. Then one day, he pronounced it "omm e lette" and miraculously a real omelet appeared. The macchiato was amazing, though I worried that the large coffee machine was going to explode each morning when it turned on. It would ferociously whistle and steam, and just about levitate from the floor.

I spent many hours at the Molla when I wasn't working with the only Speech Pathologist in the country at Yakatit Hospital, one of the few children's hospitals in Addis. Sitting outside the hotel, I always enjoyed watching the donkeys carry heavy bricks and stones across the busy and dangerous street in front of the Molla. I also loved watching the women with their white scarves and dresses walk by, usually herding a group of small children."

"Thanks, Kathie. I never stayed at the Molla, but the stories are legendary. To this day, Dr. Joe Huang talks of his fear of rats because of the Molla Hotel. How about your weekend adventures away from Addis? Kathie, do you want to start?"

"Yes, but first I need to tell you about my favorite Ethiopian friend and one of my all-time favorite people, Joseph Wondemu."

Joseph was the driver for the program. He was a small, soft-spoken, religious young man whose kindness was enormous. He picked us up each day at the Molla and took us back and forth to the hospitals. At night he put on his taxi driver hat and found us great places to eat and fun places to listen to live Ethio-jazz performances. On the weekends, he often escorted us throughout the country.

One weekend, we decided to go to Wenchi Crater Lake, 155 km west of Addis Ababa between Ambo and Welliso. Ambo was known for its mineral springs, which provided the mineral water I always drank instead of tap water or mixed with sweetened Coke.

The drive to the lake was incredibly long and dusty, as the road, like most in Ethiopia outside of the large cities (and even in areas within large cities), are constantly in disrepair. The white fine dust was so thick that Chuck and I, jammed into the back of the van, had multiple layers of scarves wrapped around our faces to help us breathe. Joseph was totally coated with the powdery road dust.

When we stopped for some drinks, Joseph turned to me and slowly said, "Katty, I think we are dying."

I responded, "Yes, Joseph, I think we are." We smiled at each other and shrugged our shoulders in amused resignation.

The lake turned out to be beautiful, a deep body of water formed by an old extinct volcano. We rode donkeys down from the top and cruised by boat on the lake. Our breathing temporarily improved while we were at the lake. The return trip was as difficult, and we ended up coughing up dust for days."

"And you Chuck?"
"I loved spending weekends outside of Addis. There were so many wonderful adventures."

I enjoyed my time in Harar, located in the southeast area of the country. Walking in the old walled city with its multicolored houses was a visual pleasure. And feeding the hyenas outside the city wall at night was unique.

Spending time in Lalibela, seeing stone churches built down from the surface into the ground, was exceptional. Kathie and I traveled there during our first trip to Ethiopia. I remember not only the churches and the crowds of white robed worshippers, but the large open-air market with colorful mounds of spices and teff (the grain used to make injera). There was one butcher stall that had the healthy lungs of a cow hanging out front as a sign that the meat was of high quality. That was quite the advertisement.

I also loved hiking in the Simien Mountains in the North with both you and Neil (Dr. Neil Schluger, the other co-director of the EATI program). Time with the Gelada baboons, the ones with the red hearts on their chests, was fascinating. Staying at the resort overlooking a Grand Canyon-like vista was special, as was our guide who informed us that we should keep a close watch for the elusive mountain chickens, which turned out to be regular free-range chickens who happened to live in the area. The story of the mountain chickens provided us with years of laughter.

> "But the most amazing adventure was with you and Neil, when you tried to kill me by climbing to the cliff churches."

Ethiopia is home to one of the oldest Christian sects. There are over 100 rock hewn churches in Northern Ethiopia, many of which sit high on mountain tops. Abuna Yemata Gah is the only operational church where you must climb a 1000-foot ledge to see it. This was the church that you, Debi, insisted we see.

The day started off easily enough. We slowly hiked up a rock path to the base of the cliff. Then the climbing began. When the guides told us to take our shoes off to make it easier to climb, I started to get nervous. But the guides, who were probably all older than me but in much better shape, took my feet and placed them into the well-worn rock indentations all the way up. I resisted looking down as we climbed higher and higher. We reached what I thought was the church and I started to relax when the priest, who had joined us, said, "Onward."

"You want me to do what?"

"Take my hand."

He guided me onto a ledge that was incredibly narrow, maybe 1-2 feet in width at most. The priest said not to worry, "God will protect you. If you fall, God will blow a wind that will bring you back to safety." There was no way I was buying that line but like so many other times in my life, I let fate carry me forward. We followed the path for 20 yards into the church opening. Inside was a most amazing sight, sixth century vibrant drawings everywhere. It really was breath taking. After all that adrenaline surge, I felt a great sense of peace and comfort within the rock walls of the church.

Going down was easier. The guides whose only English was 'left foot here and right foot here' again placed my feet into the correct foot holds. Even now, so many years later, the thrill of that adventure remains.

"That's also one of my most treasured travel experiences. Anything else you want to tell me?" The sun was setting, and I knew it was time for Debi to leave.

Kathie quickly answered, "No more stories for today, but do come back for more."

We walked Debi to the door. It had been a very pleasant visit for all of us.

We never did talk with Debi again about the early days of EATI. And after that visit, I never really spent any more significant time reminiscing about my global health career. It seemed appropriate to leave all those memories in that rock-hewn cliff church where I had found peace and comfort as so many had through the ages.

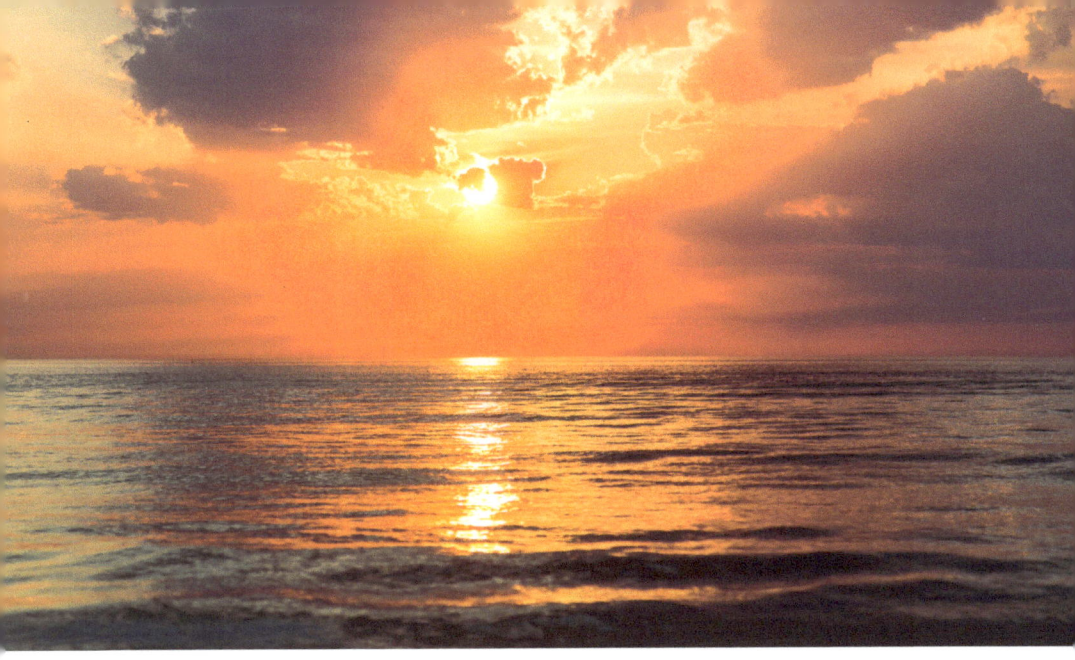

13
DIRT NAP

As I write this last chapter, I realize my own life's book is rapidly coming to a close as well. Kathie is still going strong, but my body is failing like the salmon who struggle upstream, back to their birthplace, to procreate before completely flaking into oblivion. Only I'm not procreating. Ha! (Grandma Petey would always add a "Ha!" in her letters after a sentence that humored her.)

I remember seeing those salmon on a stream outside of Juneau with Jeff when we were on our college trip to Alaska to work on the pipeline (with absolutely no skills or experience, ah youth). He actually wanted to catch one of the salmon for dinner (with his bare hands, I might add) until we saw a sign stating it was a federal offense, punishable with a sizeable fine, for interfering with spawning salmon, known by the red coloring of their backs.

> But I digress into more storytelling as I am still prone to do.
> I had always told my children that when I start peeing on the houseplants, tell me "Dad, it's time to take your dirt nap." Well, that time has arrived.
> I remember clearly when that day came for my mother.

"Chuuuuck. 103," shouted my mother, Ruth, from her bedroom across the hallway from mine in the early morning. To the uninitiated, this would make no sense. But to me, I knew my mother was conveying her weight and awaiting my orders for her furosemide diuretic dose.

At the beginning of July 2015, my 96-year-old mother came to live with Kathie and me; no not near us, but in the same house. I had not lived with my mother since I left for college at age 18; I never really thought I would again. Over the next 10 months, I served numerous roles: youngest son, concierge physician ("Why do I need another physician when I'm only going to listen to you anyway?"), supportive brother and husband, assisted living administrator, and case manager.

For six previous months, my mother had been in and out of the hospital in Boca Raton, Florida, where she had lived for over 25 years. Little did her physician know that she wasn't using her oxygen when most needed ("I didn't want to get the tubing wet in the shower") or taking her diuretic on a regular basis ("I can't be going to the bathroom all day long; that's just ridiculous!"). My mother's physician made a crucial error in assuming that she was following instructions, especially when she was getting worse despite reasonable medical interventions.

It was obvious that my mother couldn't stay in Florida; my brothers, Robert and Richard, and I couldn't keep coming down for yet another emergency hospital stay. Even my incredibly independent and "I'll never live with my children" mother understood the need to move. Walking that delicate balance between insisting on a life-changing intervention and honoring a parent's independence is difficult at best.

My brothers played the medical card which did make sense as I was the only physician in the family and a pulmonologist versed in the care of those needing supplemental oxygen. So, off my mother came to Rhode Island.

The trip itself was harrowing. My mother had both lung and heart disease and required high flow continuous supplemental oxygen. Despite having a portable battery-operated concentrator on the airplane, her oxygen saturation as measured in flight was quite low.

Why did I measure her oxygen saturation knowing that I couldn't increase the flow rate on her concentrator? And really, was I going to ask the pilot to land the plane before our descent into Providence for her low oxygen saturation? I guess I took the measurement in the hopes that it would be OK, good luck with those odds. I should have focused more on our homemade chicken sandwiches as Robert did during the trip.

My consciousness was filled with dread and anxiety during those first days. Our lives would not be the same. Our dreams of foreign travel, more time spent with adult children living elsewhere, and pursuing new interests vanished. What had I done to our sanity, our marriage?

When she first arrived, my mother was going to stay in our house just until she became more medically stable and then transition to assisted living. She had been in an independent setting in Florida, but clearly, she needed more care now. Robert and I toured several facilities, some quite nice, but we both had trouble visualizing our mother in any of them.

She would need additional full-time care due to her oxygen requirement and at considerable expense. I was convinced that I would have to field daily calls and likely make daily visits to any place she stayed. So, for "a while" we decided to keep her at our house. After all, with all her medical problems and her quite elderly age, how long could she really live—6 weeks? 3 months? But after 9 months and a fierce determination to live on, she continued with us.

For the most part, I felt like I was living on the movie set of Ground Hog Day where each day remains the same, over and over again—meals, naps, movies, CNN news, and interspersed conversations. Some days were better than others, especially when she felt well enough to bake with her aids or laugh with my son, Steve, and his girlfriend, Glenn (later his wife), during their frequent visits.

Caretaking was tough, demanding, and relentless. Even with extra help and visits from my brothers, the main responsibilities still rested with my wife and me. What a much better appreciation I developed for my wife's role as primary caregiver to our young children when they were growing up. Working in the hospital certainly had its challenges, but none as personal, emotional, or intimate as caring for a child or now an aged parent.

I gave my mother credit. She moved to a new location and a new position of less independence. She adjusted to our lifestyle, which was less formal and less materialistic than hers, and she was respectful. She praised us at times and told her friends how wonderfully we were caring for her.

She died at our house just before her 97th birthday, some 10 months after coming to live with us. She passed peacefully from an unforeseen bowel obstruction caused by a previously treated colon cancer. She lived a full and meaningful life and never stopped pushing forward, even as her body failed. In fact, her last words to me were, "Tomorrow will be a better day."

The time she spent with us was certainly trying and challenging on a daily basis. But living under the same roof provided me with an opportunity to re-work old behavior patterns, share family remembrances, and forge a new and deeper adult relationship with my mother. Kathie and I proudly provided her with last days filled with life and not focused on dying. And yes, by living with my patient, the ultimate in concierge medicine, I truly came to understand the full impact of illness and aging on both the patient and the family. May her memory be a blessing.

> And now it was my turn to take that step into the unknown.
>
> I had been reading obituaries for years, at first to keep track of my patients and then to get ideas for my own. I had written and re-written my own obituary so many times and shared many different versions with my wife. One version listed all my professional accomplishments. Another focused on my hobbies. A more recent one highlighted my marriage, children, grandchildren, and great grandchild.
>
> I loved opening phrases like "promoted to glory" and "entered into eternal life" (common ones in Africa), "cleared for final takeoff" (a pilot, of course), and "finished his work on this earth." One of my all-time favorites was for a woman who sold brassieres her whole life, "died at 97, a size 38 B."
>
> But in the end, my final version was quite short and simple.
>
> *Charles B. Sherman, age 99, died peacefully today surrounded by his wife, children, grandchildren, and great grandchild. He tried to make a difference in the world and came to realize that the love he gave and the love he received were his greatest lifetime achievements.*
>
> I knew Kathie would approve.

ACKNOWLEDGEMENTS

Over my global health career, I have worked with incredibly dedicated health care providers. Their willingness to travel long distances on their own dime to make a difference in the lives of those in need of better healthcare has always been an inspiration to me.

Special thanks to Kathie for repeatedly editing this manuscript, but more importantly for her willingness to leave her comfort zone to make so many of these trips with me. I know that I couldn't have done the work without her by my side.

ABOUT THE AUTHOR

Charles Sherman began his medical career with the AIDS epidemic and retired from clinical medicine during the COVID-19 pandemic. Over his forty-year medical career, he served as a board-certified internist, pulmonologist and critical care specialist, and as a public health epidemiologist. He was an Associate Professor of Medicine (Clinician Educator) at the Alpert Medical School of Brown University, where he was acknowledged as an award-winning clinician and teacher. He published over 60 peer-reviewed articles, editorials, and textbook chapters. For much of his career, Dr. Sherman worked on medical projects in Latin America, Africa, and Eurasia, often in leadership roles.

www.ingramcontent.com/pod-product-compliance
Lightning Source LLC
Chambersburg PA
CBHW040846240426
43673CB00013B/362